THE STRANGE DEATH OF MEDICAL ENGLAND

WILLIAM HAYES-WOOD

UK Book Publishing.com

Editing, design, typesetting and publishing by UK Book Publishing

www.ukbookpublishing.com

ISBN: 978-1-917329-93-4

THE STRANGE DEATH OF MEDICAL ENGLAND

ACKNOWLEDGMENTS

Sincere thanks to my colleagues *Dr Christopher Howard*, *Professor Harry Zeitlin* and *Professor Alistair Warren* for their wise counsel. Thanks also to *Ruth Lunn* for her overall guidance and editorial wizardry.

PROLOGUE

The title of this little book is an homage to George Dangerfield's classic work "The Strange Death of Liberal England". Dangerfield's great work had wide ranging influence over many years not only because it describes a fundamental sociopolitical change in England during the first part of the 20th century, but also because it is written in an engaging, entertaining and often amusing style. To what extent its controversial thesis is valid I cannot say, because I was not alive at the time of the events described and analysed so I am not a reliable witness to their veracity. Though I am no Dangerfield, what I can claim is that many of the key events described in this present monograph lie within my personal experience over the best part of a lifetime and thus I hope my commentary may have some value.

This book is meant to be about the medical profession – specifically its evolution over centuries and its recent demise. I could be accused of conflating the profession with the NHS (National Health Service). They are not the same thing. I do spend a great deal of time discussing the NHS. But as the NHS has evolved it and the medical profession have become so closely intertwined it can be difficult to define where one ends and the other begins. I believe this conflation is at the root of many of the problems I attempt to describe. In short, I believe the NHS is better off underpinned by an independent medical profession, free to speak truth to power, than with bonded servants fearful of their job security, working under a series of governments which have progressively tried to write out doctors from the equation.

I believe it is qualification enough to write this book in that I am a citizen of the United Kingdom whose family has used, benefited from and indeed relied upon the NHS over many years. My mother, in particular, relied on the NHS from its inception. Though this book is not about my mother, it is pertinent to say that the superb care she received from the NHS from its founding is something for which I am supremely grateful and which has influenced my thinking profoundly. Bedevilled with chronic respiratory problems since childhood, in middle and later life she received excellent care enabling her to beat breast cancer first and a decade later cancer of the cervix. A little later she underwent two knee joint replacements enabling her to walk again, and cataract surgery allowing her to see again. She lived an active life into her 90s thanks in very large part to the care she received through the NHS. Fortunately, I have not needed the care of the NHS myself to any significant extent throughout my adult life. But now in retirement the inevitable trials and tribulations of the increasing years are beginning to take their toll and, no doubt, I will require more involved care as the years go by, as indeed will we all.

Another qualification – I trust – is that I have spent a career as a doctor over more than 40 years. I stated that this book is not about my mother. And I do not want it to be about me either. Too often these days, particularly on social media, the narrative becomes more about the author than the subject. While this is something I sincerely wish to avoid, I have nevertheless chosen to include personal experiences where I believe these exemplify the point being made. My first job in the NHS was as a nursing assistant followed by medical school, then working as a junior doctor in hospitals in the north and midlands before becoming a consultant in London. I held NHS consultant appointments at no fewer than four hospitals in my career – not through any choice of wanting the moves myself – it was just that the hospitals kept getting closed down and I, and my colleagues, kept getting moved on. One of these posts involved being a clinical director and budget holder. I was also, at one stage, examiner, later senior examiner, in surgery for the London MB BS examination. In addition, I have experience of working outside the NHS as a Medical Expert Witness primarily in relation to people making claims for compensation following injury.

What points am I trying to make in this book? I am attempting to explain that health care in the UK is in danger because of a change in political philosophy at the very top of government which began 40 years ago and which successive governments have chosen to build on ever since. I explain that government realised at the outset that in order to achieve these changes it was an essential prerequisite to neutralise the power and influence of the one body which could frustrate their plans – the medical profession. I go on to describe how governments have methodically and stealthily achieved this goal and how the medical profession itself did not see what was happening until it was too late. I point out the irony of how we seem in the UK to be blundering towards the same unsatisfactory situation as pertained with medical regulation and health care in Victorian times, when "quacks" abounded – recent changes having undermined the key reforms of the 19th and 20th centuries which proved so effective in improving healthcare.

As for housekeeping matters, although the title of this book refers to England in deference to the title of Dangerfield's classic, the matters discussed apply equally to all parts of the United Kingdom as near as makes no difference. My colleagues in general practice might argue that I am concerned too much with hospital medicine. The counter argument is that hospitals are, for the most part, where doctors learn their craft before and after graduation and where they undergo higher training to become consultants in whatever specialty. Moreover, hospitals are the places where the most advanced and complicated treatments are carried out; complicated treatments are, of course, expensive and it is the expense of treatment which has worried the politicians in charge of the NHS ever since it was created; obsessively so since the time of Margaret Thatcher. I also feel obliged to point out that this book is about the medical profession – doctors – it is not concerned with developments within the dozens of other professional groups within the health service, without whose vital contribution the NHS could not exist and doctors could not function. No doubt they have their own tale to tell – and I hope they will. Re nomenclature, I refer to doctors in postgraduate training as "junior" doctors simply because this was the accepted designation until relatively recently and the case during the timeline of the majority of events described in this book. The preferred term today is "resident" doctor. Neither term is particularly appropriate in my view, but that is a discussion for another day.

Finally, this book is not written in an academic style with formal references. This is because the book has not been written for academics or professionals, but I hope it may be of interest to the general reader. If the reader wishes to explore a matter referred to in the text, a quick internet search will instantly provide enlightenment.

CHAPTER 1

The first stirrings of the winds of change

It was not until I became a consultant in 1984 that I began to take a real interest in the NHS and healthcare from the political standpoint. Until that time I had been consumed with the job which fascinated me, and which required so much reading and training of one sort and another, passing exams, research for a doctoral thesis, together with an emergency on-call commitment that would not be countenanced today. I had not really taken much notice of anything else going on because I was simply too busy getting on with the job. It is also fair to say that there was simply not the debate around the NHS in those days which was later to become apparent. While there were, of course, problems, they were not of the existential nature which they appear to be today. It is true that we did not have anything like the amazing diagnostic ability in those days which science and technology were soon to provide for us. Neither did we have the same sophistication of treatment techniques of so many sorts which are now routine. It was a simpler world, and no doubt scientific advances and the resulting increased complexity of healthcare would have required significant changes in themselves. But the issues I outline in this book are apart from all that. It is the change in the philosophy of those who rule over us which I seek to describe.

During my time as a junior doctor in the late 70s and 80s few people seriously criticised the concept of the NHS, its management or its funding. The NHS had been in existence for a generation and was already a fundamental part of national life like the monarchy or rain stopping play in the test match. The NHS was fulfilling its intended purpose of providing high quality healthcare to the population. There were of course a few radical outliers who wanted to abolish the NHS, but they were never taken seriously at the time.

Overdramatic though it might sound, something which hit me hard and left me, quite literally, with a sinking feeling in my stomach was a television programme. It came completely out of the blue and made me realise that profound change may well be imminent. During the 1980s one of the most popular politics and current affairs programmes on the TV was Weekend World. The programme was hosted by Brian Walden. Walden was an intriguing fellow. He had been a Labour MP. He was highly intelligent and a very good communicator. He was somewhat ahead of his time in that in his early years in politics he seemed very much traditional Labour, but he was swayed by Margaret Thatcher whom, quite clearly and as he admitted openly himself, he greatly admired.

He could not abide the left of labour and was sceptical of trades union influence. Though the term was not to be coined for a decade, Walden was very much a Blairite and his views exemplified the Labour Party as it was later to become under Blair and ultimately under Starmer.

The edition of Weekend World which had such an impact on me was actually a two-part special. If I recall correctly, the programmes were broadcast on consecutive Sunday evenings. The stark message of the programmes was twofold. First, the NHS could not continue in its present form because it was simply too expensive and the country could not afford it. Second, the reason spending and costs were out of control was because of doctors' profligacy. Doctors were basically spending as much as they wanted on healthcare, they were not answerable to anyone, and often they were wasting money on all sorts of equipment on a whim and expensive treatments whose value had never been proven. It was argued that the NHS had become unsustainable in its current form. This state of affairs had come about because the medical profession was out of control and the solution was to remove doctors from positions of power and influence.

I remember being staggered by this TV programme. The notion that – if there was a problem with the NHS it was because of the doctors – was an entirely new one to me. It is true that up till that time doctors were politically powerful within the NHS and, generally speaking, if they wanted something within reasonable grounds and put forward a coherent case, they would often get it. I'm not saying that the doctors were always in the right, but I have always thought, and this remains my view, that healthcare is better directed by doctors and other trained professionals working together, rather than by politicians or health insurers responsible to their shareholders.

If there were complaints about the NHS at the time of the Walden programmes – and of course there were, there always are – these would have been primarily about the delay in access to hospital outpatient clinic appointments and waiting time for admission to hospital for non-urgent procedures such as hip joint replacement or cataract surgery. In both instances, in certain parts of the country, waiting times might be measured in years rather than months. "The waiting list problem" was frequently discussed at election time and there was clamour to do something about it. It was argued that to reduce waiting lists more hospital beds, more doctors and other hospital staff were needed. In other words, more investment in the NHS – that is greater expenditure – the very thing the Walden programme was saying was impossible. They key issue flagged up was – not that the NHS was failing in its duty to provide high quality medical care – but that this was an extravagance the country could no longer afford. It cannot be overemphasised that money, not quality of care, had now become the driving force for change.

As already mentioned, Walden was generally sympathetic to Thatcher and there was no doubt in my mind that the Weekend World programmes in question were produced in cahoots with the government and putting forward government thinking. In simple terms, propaganda. A technique which was to become much more evident in UK politics thereafter. Simply put, a government would trail a policy in the media to see what the reaction was. If it was favourable, the government would feel confident to go ahead with the policy. If there was a backlash, the government would think again and might even deny the plans existed at all.

While the notion that the problem with the NHS was not lack of investment but cavalier doctors rampaging out of control left me cold, the Walden programmes didn't seem to provoke much reaction elsewhere. I don't remember any discussion of them amongst colleagues. I think I might have read a review of the programmes in the newspaper but recall no significant debate arising from it. Thus, no doubt, the government felt confident to proceed.

The really strange thing about the Walden programme, and its espousal of government thinking about the health service, was that – as previously stated – it came as a bolt out of the blue. What I did not quite realise at the time – and the penny took a while to drop – was that the government's plans to bring doctors under control were not the be-all and end-all of their plans for the health service. They were just a necessary first step to enable much more extensive changes.

Margaret Thatcher was in power as Prime Minister for eleven-and-a-half years. She had the ability to divide opinion to an extent which was almost unique. There are those who will argue that she was the greatest prime minister since the Second World War, while others will opine she was the worst thing that ever happened to our country. What everyone will agree on, however, is that Britain was a fundamentally different place in so many respects after her eleven-and-a-half years in power than it was at the beginning. In the 34 years since the end of the Second World War and Thatcher becoming Prime Minister in 1979, Labour and Conservative governments had shared power pretty much 50/50. Since Attlee, neither Labour nor Conservative had sought to bring about radical change in any aspect of national life. It was all about managing Britian's changing place in the world, no longer a great power and managing the decline of empire while trying to maintain economic and social stability at home. But Thatcher thought differently and had the strength of character which appealed at the ballot box and allowed her to force through her plans at Westminster. There were no sacred cows for Thatcher. Not public services such as water, gas and electricity or the nationalised industries such as coal and steel on which the country's industrial strength and wealth had traditionally been based. Not even the NHS. She wanted radical change throughout and she realised that certain groups had to be neutralised so as not to get in her way. Foremost amongst these were the trades unions ("the enemy within"). Through provoking deliberate confrontations with two of the traditionally most powerful unions – the miners and steelworkers – she effectively broke the power of the trades union movement. Less obvious at the time was that in taking on the NHS, Thatcher would have to deal with the doctors in much the same way as she had dealt with the miners and steelworkers. While the defeat of the unions was achieved surprisingly quickly and decisively, Thatcher was clever enough to realise that doctors and the NHS would require the long game – which she, her heirs and successors, were perfectly prepared to play.

CHAPTER 2

How did we get to where we are today?

The NHS 1948-1983

"The NHS is the closest thing the English have to a religion"
Nigel Lawson

"The institution which more than any other unites our nation"
Danny Boyle

In a book describing the evolution of the medical profession, it might seem counterintuitive to begin by describing the development and structure of the welfare state and National Health Service before that of the medical profession itself. But I contend that – within a short time of the NHS coming into being – it and the medical profession became so intimately interlinked that it is impossible to understand what is going on in one without appreciating what is going on in the other.

The evolution of the welfare state is complex and protracted, and a detailed account is far beyond the scope of this book. In brief, the first formal move towards a welfare state concerned pensions. The Liberal government elected in 1906 introduced a means-tested state old age pension. In 1909 a royal commission on the Poor Law recommended a unified medical service, but it would take nearly forty years for the vision to be realised. Unemployment insurance was introduced in 1911. In 1925 Parliament passed the Widows', Orphans' and Old Age Contributory Pensions Act.

By the end of 1942 the tide of the world war had changed decidedly. Allied (as it now was) victory was only a matter of time and thoughts were turning to rebuilding post-war Britain. It was at this juncture that William Beveridge, an economist and Liberal politician, published his famous report seeking to achieve security for all British citizens "from the cradle to the grave". A white paper entitled "A National Health Service" was produced by the Conservative Health Minister Henry Willink in 1944. Willink advocated free healthcare for all. Arising out of Beveridge came the Education Act (1944); the Family Allowance Act (1945) and the National Insurance Act (1946). Following the immediate post-war general election in 1945 the Labour Party won an overwhelming majority and in 1946 passed through parliament the National Health Act allowing for the National Health Service to come into being two years later.

The incoming Labour Prime Minister in 1945, Clement Attlee, made the fiery Welsh orator Aneurin Bevan minister of health. Consequently, it was Bevan who was charged with drawing up and steering through parliament the legislation to bring the NHS into being. It is worth remembering that – although we tend to think today of the NHS as being a Labour creation – it was, in reality, a construct of all three major parties. Beveridge was a Liberal, Willink a Conservative and Bevan Labour. A National Health Service would have come about in the years following World War Two no matter which party had been in government. What might have differed was its organisation. Bevan's vision was of one all-encompassing national organisation with no private input. The Conservatives wanted hospitals to be managed and run locally. Willink argued in parliament that managing hospitals locally would maintain the important relationship between doctor and patient. An enormous overweening, impersonal national organisation would threaten this important relationship. The Labour majority in parliament ensured that Bevan's view prevailed. In retrospect – always an advantageous standpoint – it seems to me that Willink's concerns about the importance of the doctor-patient relationship were prescient and this is something I shall return to later.

From the outset there were three guiding principles for the new health service: it should be universal, that is provide care for everyone; it should be free at the point of use; and services should be based on clinical need, not the ability to pay. There was disquiet about Bevan's proposals from two main sources: Conservative MPs in parliament and the medical profession itself. Re the former, the Labour majority in parliament was such that it didn't matter too much what the Conservatives thought. The medical profession was more tricky to handle. If doctors had refused to co-operate with the NHS it would have been finished before it even started. Bevan judged, probably correctly, that what was concerning doctors most was – not the principle of the NHS about which they were generally sympathetic – but fears about loss of their own independence and income. Hence Bevan's famous remark about doctors: "Ultimately I had to stuff their mouths with gold". Thus, he allowed consultants to carry on seeing their private patients in addition to their NHS work. Rather than paying GPs a salary, their income would be calculated on the basis of capitation, i.e. how many patients they had on their list. The doctors were won over. Bevan's negotiations with the doctors led to the notion in government that changes to the NHS would only be possible with the agreement of the medical profession, what became to be known as the "medical veto". And so, on 5 July 1948, at that time funded entirely by the state, the National Health Service came into being.

Throughout the 1950s and 60s in terms of the high quality service delivered to patients and the environment provided for healthcare professionals to work in, the new NHS was an undoubted success. The concerns which soon arose, ominous in retrospect, were about costs and funding. Somewhat naively, there had been an argument that as a properly functioning health service would lead to a healthier population, the need for medical care would gradually diminish so less money would need to be spent on health. Naive indeed. The cost to the government of the NHS in its first few years was greater than had been predicted, so, in 1952, a prescription charge of one shilling was introduced together with a charge of one pound for dental treatment in an effort to recoup some costs.

One of the more influential ministers of health was Enoch Powell who held office between 1960 and 1963. In efforts to increase efficiency, Powell reorganised hospital provision, introducing the concept of a district general hospital centralising hospital facilities on one site within a locality. Powell also began the closure of the large mental hospitals, purportedly integrating mental healthcare into the community and district general hospital. General practitioners were encouraged to group together and share higher grade premises. Doctors were perennially grumbling about their pay, so Powell set up a Royal Commission which led to the introduction of an independent review body to decide doctors' remuneration.

The 1970s was a decade of unrest in Britain. Perhaps a backlash to the "swinging sixties" with its societal liberalisation. The old certainties seemed no more. Britain joined (what was then called) the Common Market which ultimately morphed into the European Union of today. Many saw this as an abrogation of everything that Britain had stood for for centuries. The troubles in Ireland worsened, culminating in the Bloody Sunday massacre. The erstwhile minister of health, Enoch Powell, now a backbench MP, became an influential political figure in the seventies. A maverick if ever there was one, Powell had by this time been eschewed by both the Conservative and Labour parties. In 1972 he was voted by the Daily Express the most popular politician in Britain. Powell's anti-immigration and anti-Europe stances presaged the UKIP and Brexit movements, which were to become so influential a generation later.

Though there were economic crises in the seventies, most notably the war in the Middle East which led to petrol rationing, the economic lot of the average Briton actually progressed favourably during the seventies. Even though the cost of living doubled over the decade, average earnings trebled. Perhaps it was this rise in incomes, and the inflation concerns it caused the government, combined with the aggressive attitude of many of the more powerful trades unions seeking further pay rises and better working conditions, which were the most defining feature of the seventies. Miners' strikes in 1972 and 1974 led to the three-day week in an effort to conserve fuel supplies. The culmination was the "winter of discontent" in 1978/9 when relations between both public and private sector unions with the government reached rock bottom. The unions were demanding pay rises for their workers which the government claimed the country simply could not afford. There were numerous strikes leading to infamous – and somewhat overdramatic – newspaper headlines about "the dead going unburied" and "rubbish left uncollected in the streets".

The NHS was not immune from the industrial turmoil. The first group to become restive were the ancillary workers – hospital cleaners, porters, kitchen staff – who were unquestionably poorly paid. This resulted, in 1973, in the first national strike over pay in the NHS. Subsequently there were sustained campaigns by nurses and radiographers for pay rises. In 1975 junior doctors began a work to rule over poor pay and unpaid overtime. Consultants took action in defence of the privilege to admit their private patients to NHS hospitals. It could be stated that, by the end of the 1970s, industrial relations in Britain were in crisis with the NHS caught up in the turmoil. The climax came in the May 1979 general election resulting in a comfortable victory for Margaret Thatcher's Conservatives. Undoubtedly, dissatisfaction with the Labour government's handling of industrial relations was a major factor in Thatcher's victory.

For the first 30 years of its life the NHS existed in its intended form. In simple terms the NHS was the device which brokered the treatment of patients by their doctors. The government facilitated, and of course funded, this relationship and broadly speaking left the doctors to get on with it, valuing their judgement and their professional relationship with their patients. For the first 30 years of the NHS, doctors worked for their patients – as they always had – rather than for the government. Despite much grumbling and uncertainty on the part of the profession during the early negotiations with Bevan, the doctors had been won over. The doctors soon accepted that the NHS was a very good thing and had not turned them into civil servants, pen pushers or paupers. Within a short time of its founding the doctors had become amongst the most staunch supporters of the NHS.

Though it might sound contradictory to say so, just having described the unrest amongst many NHS staff during the 1970s, the first 30 years of the NHS were in my view its golden age. In terms of providing pretty much the best care possible, given the constraints of medical and scientific knowledge at the time, the NHS was unsurpassed anywhere in the world and generally recognised as such. If medical treatment existed, and a patient needed it, they would get it through the NHS, no matter who they were, high quality, and it would not cost them a penny. How can you say better than that? The concern which was arising amongst the political classes was not that the NHS did not work well in doing what it was set up to do – provide the best medical care to everyone at no charge at the point of use – but that doing so was proving increasingly expensive to the government. Moreover, as medical techniques became more advanced and sophisticated year by year, the cost rose ever upwards and the rate of increase was accelerating. It was this issue – the cost of the NHS to the government purse – which was to become the sun around which all future discussions on the future of the NHS were to revolve.

CHAPTER 3

How did we get to where we are today?

The NHS since 1983

As already described, the seventies had seen poor industrial relations throughout the country and the NHS had not been exempt largely (though not exclusively) in terms of disputes involving badly paid ancillary workers. In the 1980s, under the new Thatcher government which was to rule for the entire decade, the discontent was to emanate primarily from the doctors. In Chapter 1 I described how shocked I had been by the Weekend World TV programme which argued that the fundamental problem with the NHS was that the doctors were basically running it and spending money as they pleased on unproven techniques, wasting money without any oversight or control. (In fact, studies had shown that compared with other healthcare systems elsewhere in the world the NHS was strikingly efficient – but a determined politician never lets the truth get in the way of a favoured policy.)

Thatcher's approach became known as managerialism. She appointed Sir Roy Griffiths to report on the management and budget structure of the NHS. Griffiths was a businessman from the private sector who had been director of a company producing weedkiller and then a director of the Sainsbury's supermarket chain. Coming from such a background it was clear that Thatcher expected Griffiths to look at the NHS as a private sector company rather than as a state-funded organisation providing essential services based on the citizens' requirements. Of course, the overriding duty of a private sector business such as a chemical company or supermarket is to provide monetary profit for its shareholders, a concept which is meaningless to a nationalised provider of healthcare. Moreover, if the company fails to make money it can be wound up, dissolved, cease to exist. Another concept inapplicable to the NHS.

Griffiths reported in 1983, the year before I was appointed to my first consultant post in London. There is no doubt that in those days doctors as a profession, particularly consultants working in London teaching hospitals, had significant political clout. The initial rumblings, and the eventual turmoil, instigated by Thatcher were more readily apparent in London because the capital had traditionally absorbed more than its fair share of healthcare resource. The government argued that resources should be spread more equitably across the country. It was difficult to argue against this notion. As it turned out, the government of the day found this inequality in resource a useful smokescreen to hide a more cynical agenda. It turned out the intention was not to be a levelling up of resource outside London but levelling down of resource within London. But the PR was slick.

Griffiths stated that when it came to management and accountability in the NHS as he found it in 1983, basically there was none. Not in any meaningful fashion, at least. Decisions were taken on a consensus basis with various interest groups each sticking their oar in. Traditionally the most powerful of these groups was the doctors. Griffiths recommended setting up an NHS Management Board at national level at arm's length from the government to decide priorities. He recommended general managers be appointed on high salaries (comparable to those paid in the private sector) to take overall charge and manage budgets. These managers would be selected from private industry, the civil service, current hospital administrators or wherever. Griffiths stated that doctors should be closely involved with the new management process. Counter-intuitively, this was a master stroke in undermining the influence of the doctors. They became bound up in corporate decision making, unable to act independently, crucially ending the "doctors' veto" of which previous generations of health ministers had been so wary.

Had such a change as proposed by Griffiths been recommended during the first decade of the NHS's existence it is unlikely to have prevailed. Simply, the doctors would have seen it as an attempt to curtail their influence – which it was – and would have rejected it. Likely the government would have backed down rather than risked confrontation with the medical profession. All the senior doctors would have had long experience of practising their craft without the NHS and would have likely threatened to go back to the status quo. But the difference at the time of the Griffiths report was that – whereas previously the NHS had needed the doctors more than the doctors had needed the NHS – the situation was now dramatically reversed. The great majority of doctors were now entirely dependent on the NHS to function. Indeed, they knew no other system. (When I was first appointed as a consultant in 1984 this was to a health authority in London comprising two large general hospitals and several smaller specialist hospitals. The number of consultants working in the group was in excess of a hundred. Of all these senior doctors, only one, a general surgeon whose retirement was months away, had qualified before the NHS came into being. Thus, no doctor in the hospital group, bar one, had any experience of work before the NHS.)

The next key event was heralded by an interview Mrs Thatcher gave to the BBC in the run up to the 1987 general election. Thatcher was asked whether she trusted the NHS enough to use it herself. The prime minister replied:

"I, along with something like five million other people [have private health insurance] to enable me to go into hospital on the day I want; at the time I want, and with a doctor I want."

Following her (third) general election victory Thatcher gave an interview on the BBC Panorama programme in 1988 announcing that a further review of the NHS was imminent. Again, her government's concern was – not that it was not doing a good job in providing healthcare – but that the NHS was simply too expensive. The outcome of the review was published in a white paper "Working for Patients" in 1989. In summary the paper recommended:

- Money in the NHS should follow the patient by the introduction of an internal market. GPs should become fundholders. It was argued that this would improve quality and efficiency.
- Hospitals should be self-managed service providers (later becoming trusts).
- Private health insurance should be promoted by tax relief.

Out of this arose "The National Health Service and Community Care" Act of 1990. An internal market for the NHS was introduced whereby GPs were encouraged to become the fundholders. The hospitals ("providers") became trusts. Health authorities ceased to manage hospitals but could purchase care from them, not necessarily those within their own area but from wherever in the country they chose, theoretically increasing competition.

Relations between the government and the medical profession deteriorated further during the 1980s. The various management and accounting reforms introduced under the Conservative government antagonised much of the medical profession. Their influence on the workings of the NHS had been much diminished and the medical veto abolished. At the end of the decade doctors were openly hostile to government reforms and vocal in criticising them. It is ironic that the medical profession – somewhat wary of the NHS when it had first been set up by the Attlee government in 1948 – had morphed into some of the strongest supporters of state-run medicine and fiercest opponents of market based economics being introduced into the NHS. Such was the achievement of Margaret Thatcher.

Following the fall of Thatcher, the Conservative government limped on for a surprisingly long time under John Major. During the Major government there was relatively little in the way of NHS reform. By the 1997 general election there were virtually no wheels left on the Conservative wagon, allowing Tony Blair's "New Labour" to sweep to a massive victory. Labour would remain in power for the next 13 years. One of Labour's promises prior to the election was to stop Conservatives' (alleged) plans to privatise the NHS. In a speech shortly after his 1997 election victory, Blair stated that his government would abandon the NHS internal market and fund holding. He promised to replace the internal market with "integrated care", putting doctors and nurses in charge of deciding priorities. But in the years ahead Blair did not abolish the internal market. He strengthened it.

There is no doubt that investment in the NHS did increase significantly under Blair. There were sustained efforts to improve clinical and managerial governance and reduce waste. The main thrust of the New Labour government was – while leaving healthcare free at the point of use – to encourage use of the private sector. There was no attempt to reverse the outsourcing of ancillary services to private companies, much to the disappointment of the trades unions. Thus, by the time the Labour left government in 2010, there was more private sector involvement in the NHS than there had been in 1997 when it came to power.

The major contribution of the Blair government to private sector involvement in the NHS was via the Private Finance Initiative, or PFI. The scheme was politically advantageous in that it was not the sort of thing that a patient undergoing healthcare would be directly aware of, neither did it directly affect the doctor-patient relationship. PFI was actually introduced by the Conservative government in 1992 but used sparingly at first. But the Blair government expanded PFI significantly. Put simply, if the government wanted to build a new hospital, rather than stumping up the money itself it would commission a private consortium of banks and financiers to carry out the development. Once built, the consortium would be responsible for the cost of maintenance and cleaning of the building thereafter. The advantage to the government was that the money necessary for the initial build did not appear as a capital cost in the accounts and was therefore in line with the neoliberal holy grail of not increasing public expenditure. Rather, the government would pay back the private consortium over a period of time – with, of course, interest. The scheme was a bit like buying a car. One can either buy a car costing £10,000 by paying cash, giving outright ownership. Or one can buy the car on hire purchase paying monthly repayments over a typical period of three years – with interest. The disadvantage of hire purchase for a car is that you end up paying a lot more in total for the car than a cash purchase because of the interest charges. So it is with the government financing hospitals through PFI. But the ultimate cost to the government of building a hospital under PFI is massively greater in terms of interest payments than the analogy of the car. For example, in 2012, new buildings were opened by Bart's Hospital in London funded by PFI. The cost of the construction was £1.15 billion. The deal was over 35 years, at the end of which the government would have paid back, in regular instalments, a total of over £7 billion. These deals are generally much more lucrative to the private companies involved than is the case for a hire purchase company financing cars or a building society offering a home mortgage. In the most egregious example, the PFI consortium has made a 70% annual profit.

The Labour government fell in 2010 to be replaced initially by a Conservative-led coalition with the Liberal Democrats. After 2015 this became a majority Conservative government apart from a brief hiccup post-Brexit when the government required support from the DUP (Democratic Unionist Party). Andrew Lansley became secretary of state for health, and his policy ideas culminated in the Health and Social Care Act of 2012. This came to be regarded as the most complex, radical, wide-ranging and controversial piece of legislation in the history of the NHS. It was opposed by almost all healthcare professional groups, one of the most consistent criticisms being that the proposed reforms were incomprehensible. The most visible measure was setting up a new management board called NHS England to manage the entire NHS supposedly independent of the government department of health.

Even Lansley's own colleagues in government were confused. One government insider is quoted as saying "*No one apart from Lansley had a clue what he was really embarking on. Certainly not the Prime Minister*". A review of the bill by leading counsel concluded "the duty to provide a national health service would be lost... it replaces a 'duty to provide' with a 'duty to promote'".

Somewhat later Lansley himself said that the point of the Act was to "*stop the NHS from being a political football*" but it is difficult to work out how his Act was supposed to achieve this. The details of the Act are far too complex to be detailed here, but a summary of the effects of the 2012 Act published by the King's Fund stated:

- The reforms resulted in top-down reorganisation of the NHS, which was distracting and damaging.

- The reforms resulted in greater marketisation of the NHS.

- New systems of governance and accountability were complex and confusing.
- The absence of system leadership was increasingly problematic when the NHS needs to undertake major service changes.

Lansley's successor as secretary of state for health Jeremy Hunt said of the Act: "The idea of lots of competing foundation trusts and payment by results works well when you have in your mind that most of the work the NHS does will be single episode elective care, but when you're dealing with complex patients who are going in and out of the system a lot those structures prove not to be fit for purpose."

Nick Timmins (a leading healthcare journalist) wrote in 2018 that the legislation was a failure in its own terms. Choice and competition had turned out not to be the driving principles of the NHS. "*Political micro-management*" and "*excessive bureaucratic and political control*" had not disappeared. David Benbow (school of law, Sheffield University) wrote in 2020 that the legislation did not extend patient choice as envisaged but led to an increasing amount of the NHS budget being diverted to private providers. Over the period 2019-2022 a series of measures was enacted by government which, without formally passing a new act, effectively abolished the major tenets of the Lansley legislation. A report written by the surgeon and independent peer Lord Darzi in 2024 concluded "*The Health and Social Care Act of 2012 was a calamity without international precedent – it proved disastrous. The result of the disruption was a permanent loss of capability from the NHS... rather than liberating the NHS, as it had promised, the Health and Social Care Act 2012 imprisoned more than a million NHS staff in a broken system for the best part of a decade*".

Of rather more direct importance to doctors than the beleaguered 2012 Act was the dispute which began in 2015 between junior doctors and the health secretary Jeremy Hunt. The main grumble of the junior doctors concerned pay. Their salaries had not kept pace with inflation, so they were increasingly worse off year by year. The unhappiness was not solely due to pay, however; there were also concerns about working conditions and career prospects. Hunt's pay offer was judged inadequate and it was pointed out that doctors working the longest hours would actually receive a pay cut if Hunt's plans were agreed. The culmination in 2016 was the first doctors' strike in 40 years. Hunt was intransigent and threatened to impose a new contract. The dispute grumbled on and was not finally resolved until the new Labour government came into power in 2024, with junior doctors accepting a 22% pay rise over two years. Since the beginning of this dispute and its eventual settlement, the junior doctors had taken industrial action on no fewer than 11 occasions.

Though their dispute was overshadowed by the prolonged dispute of their junior colleagues, the senior doctors were also in dispute with the government over matters of contract and pay. Consultants took industrial action, which was eventually settled in 2024 shortly before the fall of the Conservative government, at which time the resident doctors' dispute was still festering on.

Quite what the plans of the Labour government elected in 2024 are for the NHS and medical professions remains, at the time of writing, to be seen. The new health secretary Wesley Streeting has, however, announced that NHS England will be abolished, bringing the NHS once again under direct government control. It looks likely, therefore, that yet another major reorganisation of the NHS is imminent. The old aphorism concerning deckchairs and the RMS Titanic spring to mind.

CHAPTER 4

How did we get to where we are today?

Regulation of the Medical Profession 1858-2003

As regards the medical profession, one has to go back a long way to find out how we got here because the evolution has continued over centuries. It is helpful to focus on the Medical Act of 1858. The point of this Act was to regulate the medical profession and provide a register of properly qualified practitioners so that someone seeking medical advice could be confident that a practitioner was properly trained and qualified. The situation before 1858 was complex and confusing and had been for centuries. There were no fewer than 19 organisations purporting to produce a register of trained practitioners. Prior to the 1858 Act, there were basically three main groups of medical practitioner: the physician, the surgeon and the apothecary. The physician was at the top of the pecking order. He (there were no shes) was a graduate of Oxford or Cambridge universities and would equate to the consultant or specialist of today. In recognition of their great learning, they were allowed to call themselves "Doctor", unlike surgeons or apothecaries. Physicians would treat internal diseases by the administration of "physic" or medicine, hence the name physician. In 1518 physicians in London had formed themselves into the College of Physicians, which granted licences to practise medicine to those enrolled on its books. Physicians made up a small proportion of medical practitioners, were almost exclusively confined to London, and their fees were out of the reach of ordinary folk. Therefore, the apothecary was probably the most likely port of call for most people. Their scope of practice was somewhere between that of a modern GP and a pharmacist. Their training was by apprenticeship to an established apothecary. The Society of Apothecaries was one of the longstanding livery companies of the City of London and in 1815 was awarded the power by act of parliament to grant its own licence, covering England and Wales, following a five-year apprenticeship to an established apothecary.

Surgeons, like apothecaries, had been traditionally trained by apprenticeship. Surgeons dealt with the conditions which physicians and apothecaries did not, such as setting broken bones, suturing wounds, amputations, drainage of abscesses and so on. The profession had evolved from a motley collection of barber-surgeons, bone setters and dentists. In 1800 the College of Surgeons was formed in London. No surgeon could practise within London without having passed the College's exam. Of course, this left much of the greater part of the country outwith the reach of the London College's influence.

You can see already that the College of Physicians, the College of Surgeons and the Society of Apothecaries could each offer licences to practise their own brand of medicine but their influence was largely confined to London. Of the multiple organisations offering licences of various sorts there was one body which could and did award licences to practise in local areas anywhere in England. This was – unlikely though it might first appear today – the Church of England. In fact, the Church was the major organisation issuing licences to practise medicine in England for hundreds of years. Its sanction to do so was granted by an Act of Parliament of 1511. Each bishop in his diocese had the right to grant a licence to applicants he considered sufficiently well qualified and upstanding. Quite what criteria the cleric took into account in awarding the licence is not clear.

The church's role in regulating medical practice at the time it was called upon to do so was not so daft as it might seem to us today. The fact is that – outside London or the university cities (of which there were only two in England, Oxford and Cambridge, until the University of Durham was founded in 1832) – by far the best educated people in any locality were the clerics. Consequently, there is a logic in their authority to "examine" (in the loosest sense of the word) and grant medical licences on behalf of their community. One curiosity of this system was that the church licences applied only to the diocese in which they were issued. A licence issued by the Bishop of Chester would not apply in the neighbouring diocese of Lichfield and *vice versa*. These were not licences to practise nationally.

The Medical Act of 1858 (*An Act to Regulate the Qualifications of Practitioners in Medicine and Surgery*) was monumentally important in the regulation of medical practice in England. As already stated, before the Act there were no fewer than 19 different organisations publishing their own register claiming to authorise competence as a medical practitioner of one sort or another. For the first time the Act brought together all those deemed to hold proper, professional medical qualifications on a single national register so patients would know if they were seeing a properly trained professional or not. Importantly, those not professionally qualified – colloquially known as "quacks" – could not claim to be registered medical practitioners. To falsely do so became a criminal offence. The 1858 Act, more than anything else, marked the birth of the medical profession in England as we were to recognise it for the next 150 years.

In order to draw up and maintain the medical register the General Medical Council (*General Council of Medical Education and Registration of the United Kingdom*) usually abbreviated to GMC was brought into being as a statutory body. Within the GMC the office of registrar was created to oversee the medical register. Over the years there have been a number of amendments to the provisions of the 1858 Act – hardly surprising given the changes in science and society since 1858. These have largely been related to fitness to practise issues and undergraduate education. However, the two fundamentals of the Act persisted and remained in force for 150 years or so. The fundamentals being, of course, to maintain a register of properly qualified doctors and to remove from the register those whose practice, educational standard or behaviour failed to meet the proper requirement. Second, that the compilation of the register and the supervision of standards and safe medical practice should be overseen by the GMC as a body which was independent of the government of the day.

Initially the GMC was managed by a council of more than 100 members, all doctors, elected by the profession itself. Over time the council has been gradually reduced in size and the concept of self-regulation has fallen into disrepute so that lay members were introduced onto the board. The essence of the GMC was gradually eroded from its original concept, piece by piece, bit by bit, the tipping point coming under the Blair government in 2003.

CHAPTER 5

How did we get to where we are today?

Regulation of the Medical Profession since 2003

While the governing council of the GMC – as instigated by the 1858 Act – remains today, it is elementally different in its structure. Currently, the governing council of the GMC consists of 12 members, six of whom are doctors and six of whom are not. Before 2003 doctors themselves had elected their own representatives onto the council, but in 2003 this democratic privilege was removed from them after 147 years. (Doctors were not, however, relieved of the privilege of having to pay a hefty annual subscription to fund the Council and its activities and thus remain on the register – in effect a tax.) All members of the GMC, whether lay or medical, are now appointed by the privy council. In other words, appointed by the government. This change in 2003, in my opinion, marked the tipping point when the medical profession gave up on itself; after this point the profession finally acknowledged its subservience to the government of the day. The long-held concept of an independent self-governing profession was gone. An ominous development.

The 2003 changes, in effect, give the government control of the GMC – and thereby regulation of the medical profession and (although the government would no doubt vigorously deny this) *de facto* control of the medical profession. This is in direct contrast to the situation ever since the 1858 Act and to Aneurin Bevan's assertion at the foundation of the NHS that he was not going to turn the medical profession into government employees. But the fact is the medical profession is no longer the independent profession it once was.

Perhaps the most egregious appointment to the GMC took place under the Conservative government in 2016. The secretary of state for health, Jeremy Hunt, had been involved in an acrimonious, drawn-out dispute with junior doctors, wanting to alter their contract, which would have meant that juniors working the longest hours would receive a pay cut. Industrial action resulted and the debate was distinctly bad tempered all round. The Director of Acute Care and Workforce at the Department of Health working closely with Hunt at the time of the junior doctors' dispute was one Charlie Massey. In 2016 Massey was slotted into post as Chief Executive/Registrar of the GMC, in effect the main man. Despite Freedom of Information requests concerning the precise details of his appointment, these have not been forthcoming. Dr Phil

Hammond wrote in Private Eye at the time: *"The GMC is supposed to be an independent medical regulator, so the appointment of one of Hunt's stooges who is overseeing contract imposition to the most senior GMC role gives doctors grave cause for concern. The GMC has the power to strike off striking doctors and to remove trainees from trusts, if they are felt not to meet training standards, which are themselves decided by the GMC. The GMC could in theory influence contract imposition and hospital closures, which is why its independence from government, and appearance of independence is vital. So why appoint Massey?"* Why indeed. One consequence of this is the doctors are much more fearful of speaking out, on behalf of patients and the NHS, as they realise their comments may be perceived as unhelpful towards government policy on health.

Another ominous change relates to the GMC's acceptance of the government's decision (despite the profession as a whole being decidedly against) that – besides keeping a unique register of qualified doctors – the GMC should start registering two new grades of para medical practitioner, that is PAs and AAs. A PA is a Physician Associate, and an AA is an Anaesthetic Associate. So the GMC is now (since 2024) maintaining a register of people who are not doctors, have not trained as doctors and are not qualified to be doctors or to call themselves doctors. These non-doctors are given a GMC registration number akin to that which the GMC gives qualified doctors. In other words, the GMC is doing today exactly what it was originally set up to specifically prevent – that is, registering practitioners who are not trained as doctors, who have never been to medical school or obtained a degree in medicine. This decided perversity is something else I go into in greater detail later, in Chapter 7. One telling curiosity of the GMC today is that it has chosen to unburden its staff from reliance on the NHS for their own medical care. The GMC now provides all of its employees with private health insurance. It is difficult to know what to make of this but no explanation I can think of casts the GMC or the NHS in a particularly good light. What is certain, however, is that this privilege is paid for by the subscriptions of ordinary doctors who receive no such benefit themselves. Doctors' hefty subscriptions are supposed to finance the production and maintenance of a legal document, the medical register, not provide valuable freebies for GMC staff.

Another avenue which the GMC has chosen to go down relates to PR – or propaganda or spin – call it what you will. One of the best examples relates to the published review in 2016 of the consultation concerning the implementation of the GMC's new appraisal/revalidation procedure for doctors. Comments from the profession itself, who had undergone the procedure, were almost wholly negative and dismissive, the basic criticism being the procedure was not fit for purpose. Yet an independent person reading the report would be led to believe it was an outstanding success. The spin was quite remarkable. Similar spin has been seen in relation to senior appointments to the GMC and discussions surrounding the introduction of Physician Associates. The constant theme in these dealings, or so it seems to me, is the avoidance of commenting on government policy and discouraging doctors from voicing criticism of the government. One could be forgiven for thinking that the GMC now sees its role as protecting the government from any disquiet the doctors may wish to express. But there again, one has to remember that knighthoods and DBEs may be at stake.

The GMC has taken careful note of the growth and importance of social media. Dr Rachel Clarke, a palliative care specialist, exposed the GMC as having hired social media experts to digitally snoop on doctors' social media posts to see what criticisms they were making about the GMC and "*shape [its] subsequent strategy*". Big Brother is watching you.

There can be no doubt that the medical profession currently holds the GMC in low esteem. Perhaps the strongest criticism the medical profession has of the GMC relates to the notion that – when things go wrong because of inadequacies in the system – the GMC strives to throw the relevant doctor under the bus rather than highlighting the deficiencies, stress and strain, under which doctors are often forced to work in the NHS. No case indicates this better than that of Dr Bawa-Garba.

Dr Bawa-Garba was a registrar in paediatrics (children's medicine) in Leicester. Tragically, on the day in question, a young child died and there were undoubted errors in his management which contributed to the death. As the doctor looking after him, Dr Bawa-Garba was prosecuted for involuntary manslaughter and, under the judge's direction, found guilty by a majority of 10-2. She was given a two-year suspended prison sentence and referred to the MPTS (Medical Practitioners Tribunal Service).

On the day in question Dr Bawa-Garba was working as the sole doctor in charge of the Children's Assessment Unit at a major NHS hospital. She was new to the hospital and had received no induction. There was no supervising consultant available and, owing to staff shortages, she was covering the work of two other doctors. There was an IT systems failure in the hospital so the results of important blood tests were not available. There was additional confusion regarding patients being moved about the ward and prescribed medication because of poor communication between various staff. That day, Dr Bawa-Garba worked a 13-hour shift without a break. In other words, the system in which Dr Bawa-Garba was forced to work was simply not fit for purpose and she was working under a great deal of strain without proper support. It is hardly surprising that errors are made in such circumstances. The court's judgement was widely criticised. It is worth noting that – prior to this incident – Dr Bawa-Garba's career record had been impeccable. There was a feeling in some quarters that she had been made a scapegoat for a failing system.

Any issues concerning the court's judgement apart, the response of the GMC was subject to even greater criticism and greatly undermined what faith the medical profession still had in the GMC. As stated above, following the court verdict Dr Bawa-Garba was referred to the MPTS who recommended that she be suspended from the medical register for a period of 12 months. The MPTS was set up through the Medical Act of 1983 as a body separate from the GMC to assess a doctor's fitness to practise. Obviously, a conviction of manslaughter raises questions about a doctor's fitness to practise and hence Dr Bawa-Garba's referral to the MPTS was inevitable. The MPTS considered Dr Bawa-Garba's actions to be neither "*deliberate or reckless*" and decided that she did not "*pose a continuing risk to patients*", therefore erasure (i.e. permanent removal) from the medical register would be disproportionate. She was therefore suspended from practice for 12 months. The GMC was unhappy with this decision and appealed it to the divisional court on the basis that, in the interests of public confidence, a conviction of manslaughter should lead to permanent erasure from the medical register. The court found in favour of the GMC and Dr Bawa-Garba's name was erased from the register.

Dr Bawa-Garba appealed this decision to the high court. The high court threw out the divisional court's ruling on the basis that the criminal court and the MPTS fulfilled different functions. It was ruled that the tribunal was entitled to take the systemic failings of the hospital and others into account when deciding sanction, in the same way as the criminal court when passing sentence. It was pointed out that the GMC's own ordnances clearly outline that the purpose of fitness to practise proceedings is not to punish the doctor a second time. Therefore, if the doctor presents no danger to the public – as Dr Bawa Garba did not – their career should not be sacrificed in order to satisfy a demand for blame and punishment. Consequently, Dr Bawa Garba's name was restored to the register after 12 months as the MPTS had originally ruled. Arising out of this case the Williams Report (2018) recommended that the GMC be stripped of its right to appeal MPTS cases.

The fundamental reason for the concern which the GMC's decision to appeal raised within the medical profession was that the GMC appeared to accept that the unsatisfactory, failing conditions within the NHS in which doctors were condemned to work should be tolerated as the norm. In other words, if doctors were unable to practise safe medicine in an unsatisfactory, sometimes dangerous, system of healthcare in which they had to work, then that was their bad luck. In other words, it was the doctor who had to bear the responsibility for errors made consequent upon the failings of the system in which they worked, not the system itself. This case therefore represents a classic example of the GMC deciding its responsibility is to avoid criticism of the system – the NHS, government health policy – at the expense of the doctor and ultimately of the patient. The GMC saw its role as protector of government health policy, in preference to that of the unbiased arbiter of the doctor's performance or the protector of the patient. A wholly perverse state of affairs.

CHAPTER 6

Student funding and postgraduate training in the Blair era

"It really is hard for anybody not in medicine and paying close attention, to fully understand how badly this generation of UK trainees is being treated and how profound the effects will be"
Prof Mark Toshner

There are two main considerations in the funding of undergraduate studies leading to a degree in medicine: payment to the university to take part in the course and the cost of day-to-day living expenses for the student. The former is the tuition fee and the latter the maintenance grant or loan.

Following World War Two and the social revolution brought about in its aftermath by the Attlee Labour government, most students going up to university had their tuition fees paid by the local authority. This was eventually formalised by statute in 1962, after which university education was free for all students. The 1962

Education Act also directed local authorities to pay a maintenance grant to university students, which did not have to be repaid. The grant was means-tested. The grant was sufficient for a student to live on during the university terms. When I went up to university in 1971, my grant worked out at £10.10 per week during term. My parents paid a small top-up. Astounding as this sounds today a little over £10 per week allowed me to pay for my accommodation, food, bus fares etc. I could not tell you what the university tuition fee was because it was paid directly by the local authority to the university and was of no concern to me. I was one of the lucky ones – something I now know and appreciate. But it just seemed normal at the time. Nobody questioned it. The freedom from financial worry and hardship which my generation of undergraduates had taken as the norm was to be denied to future generations of medical students and doctors. Why? The only explanation I can fathom is that the changes reduced government expenditure and opened up aspects of medical training to the private sector. Once again, the driving force behind the government's changes had nothing to do with improving the service provided to patients or better trained doctors. It was all about reducing government spending and dangling the carrot of reduced taxes to the electorate.

As it is the most direct concern of students on a continuing day-to-day basis, let's look at the changes to the maintenance aspect first. Inevitably, the process of change began when Thatcher came to power. A consistent theme of the Thatcher government which was in power throughout the 1980s was to reduce state spending on just about everything and privatise anything it could. With inflation continuing to take its toll, rather than increasing the value of the student grant to compensate, the government decided to offer top-up loans to students, to be paid back after graduation when they were earning money. The Student Loans Company was set up in 1990 and a typical loan was in the order of £400. As time went on the value of the student maintenance grant was gradually reduced under successive governments so that by 2016 it had been effectively abolished. Concurrent with the phasing out of the maintenance grant was an increase in the amount which students could borrow as a loan. So, gradually over the course of a quarter century, student grants were phased out in favour of student loans. The amount which can be borrowed by a student today (2024/25) for maintenance is £10,227 at an interest rate of 3% over RPI. (This figure is for students studying outside London. The figure is a little higher for those at university in the capital.) The loan, and interest, are repayable when the graduate starts earning over the threshold (for some students this is £25,000 per year, for other students it is £27,295). The monthly repayment goes up as income increases so those on incomes which remain low pay a smaller amount, which, of course, means the loan takes longer to pay off and interest continues to be accrued.

Turning to tuition fees, it was the Labour government under Thatcher's heir, Tony Blair, who made students responsible for paying their own tuition fees through the Teaching and Higher Education Act of 1998. Tuition fees of £1,000 per academic year were introduced and further student loans were made available to cover the fee. Tuition fees have risen over time and now stand at £9,250 (increasing to £9,535 from September 2025).

Through a freedom of information request in 2024 a BBC journalist established that something like 1.8 million people in the UK are now in £50,000 or more student debt and over 60,000 owe more than £100,000. Some 50 people owe in excess of £200,000. But ex-students can take some comfort that if the loan has still not been repaid after 40 years, it will be written off. Because of the prolonged and practical nature of their course, the student debts incurred by doctors tend to be towards the upper end of the scale.

The requirement for doctors to undergo further compulsory training following graduation did not exist at the start of the NHS. As soon as you received your diploma on graduating from medical school and, a couple of weeks later, received confirmation that your name had been added to the medical register, that was it. You could go straight into general practice. In 1953 a further year's training in hospitals after graduation became compulsory (pre-registration house officer) and only after this was full registration granted. So you had to wait another year after getting your degree before you could work outside hospital unsupervised and become a GP. This remained the situation when I graduated from medical school in the 1970s. You could go straight into general practice and become a GP principal as soon as you had completed your house officer year in hospital. No further training or qualification was required. At least two of my classmates did exactly this. In both instances their parents were established GPs and my colleagues simply joined the family business. They were the exceptions, however. Almost all of my generation of young doctors chose to gain further experience in hospital posts before choosing their final career within medicine. In 1981 a further year's training became compulsory before entering general practice. A year later this extra training requirement was increased to three years. Currently, GP training is not complete until a minimum of five years after graduation. As regards general practice at least there is no doubt that on entering general practice today the principal or salaried GP is better trained and more experienced than was the case in the early years of the NHS, bringing about obvious benefit to patients, and this is to be applauded. It is questionable whether the same benefit has been apparent in the training of specialists and consultants over the past 20 years.

For those choosing a career in hospital medicine in the early years of the NHS, the progression to consultant was by no means so prescriptive and inflexible as it is today. This is not to say, however, that those in training gained less experience in those days than consultants appointed today – quite the opposite in fact. The difference was the specialist in training was much freer to decide in which areas and which hospitals he or she wished to gain experience. Until the 1980s a hospital appointments committee could appoint whoever it deemed suitable to a consultant post provided they held full registration with the GMC. In practice, appointees would have acquired considerable experience in a variety of junior or resident posts before appointment. They would most likely have obtained postgraduate qualifications as well, though this was not inevitable. When I was first appointed a consultant, two of the senior consultants at my hospital who had been originally appointed in the 1970s had no postgraduate qualification, just their primary degree. (I should perhaps add that both were able to fulfil their consultant roles admirably and in one case with distinction.)

For the first 50 years of the NHS, junior doctors were free to apply for any job they wished in any hospital. The hospital appointment committee was free to appoint whoever it wanted to a training post. In this less rigid system most young doctors did not make a final career choice until some years after graduation. The norm was to work at several jobs in hospital, after the first compulsory year gaining general experience which, in itself, would be valuable whatever career was eventually chosen. Whether ultimately pursuing a career in general practice, paediatrics, laboratory medicine, public health or whatever. Doctors devised their own training programmes to suit their own preferences and requirements. Though my own postgraduate qualification FRCS – Fellow of the Royal College of Surgeons – is in general surgery (which was all there was at the time for aspiring surgeons anyway, specialist fellowships not yet having been introduced), I worked as a junior doctor in a variety of specialities typically in six-month blocks to gain a wide experience. Besides (obviously) general surgery, these included orthopaedics, plastic surgery, thoracic surgery, paediatrics, paediatric surgery, accident and emergency, and anaesthetics/intensive care. Such a wide hinterland prior to becoming a consultant is unusual today. Training was very much practical based, on the job, in all meaningful respects an apprenticeship learning the skills from one's established seniors. Standards of postgraduate training were overseen by the medical royal colleges (in other words by committees of senior doctors, not by government or NHS managers). Each specialty was associated with a particular college. Each college offered its own examination to accede to membership or fellowship of the college. Confusingly, perhaps, becoming a Member of the Royal College of Physicians or a Fellow of the Royal College of Surgeons did not in itself mean you could immediately become a consultant. The exam was a staging post in the journey, more a box successfully ticked, allowing you to carry on with further training to complete the journey sufficiently to impress a consultant appointment committee to give you a job several years later down the line.

A consultant physician, surgeon or gynaecologist, on appointment, generally had significantly more experience of their practical craft under the old system than is the case today. An article by Ian Griggs in the Independent in 2007 noted that prior to the Blair government changes described below, the number of hours clinical training before becoming a constant averaged out at 21,000. Following the Blair government changes, the number of hours required to train a consultant had dropped to 6,000.

Just as with the funding of medical training, the Blair government was to bring about sweeping changes to the training of junior doctors to enable them to progress to senior positions within the NHS. The Labour government led initially by Tony Blair was elected in 1997 and remained in power until 2010. Blair himself was prime minister for the first ten years before giving way to Gordon Brown. Within a short time of coming to power, Blair promised a major shake-up in all aspects of the NHS. The proposals were outlined in a document entitled NHS Plan 2000, the contents of which were generally welcomed in large part because the plan included major financial investment in the NHS, something which had noticeably been lacking in the numerous other programmes for change over previous decades. It has to be said that Blair was true to his word on the investment and it did take place. It is also true that – as so often happens in politics – plans do not always bring about the hoped-for benefit even when introduced with the best intentions. The changes brought about in medical training and career structure under Blair's premiership were radical, even impacting on the sort of person who was able to become a doctor.

Following on from NHS Plan 2000 there was to be a major revamp in the postgraduate training of doctors introduced in 2005 as Modernising Medical Careers (MMC). The stated aim of the modernisation plan was to "*improve patient care by improving medical education with a transparent and efficient career path for doctors*". Of course, the phrase "improving patient care" is essential preliminary spin put on any proposed change to healthcare. It implies that, at the end of it all, the patient would benefit from better trained doctors. In reality, this claim is questionable, as applied to the training of hospital consultants at least. The changes had the effect of reducing the time spent in training as evinced by the Griggs figures quoted earlier in this chapter. It is difficult to see how a sweeping reduction in training can produce a better consultant at the end of it all. How is a consultant with substantially reduced training in a better position to provide patient care?

The extent to which the MMC changes formalised training programmes for postgraduate doctors was revolutionary. Career paths now had to be chosen at an early stage and once the decision had been made it was difficult to switch careers. As regards general practice, the length of training required before being issued with a Certificate of Completion of Training (CCT) was much in line with the system before Blair took office. It was training in hospital specialties leading to consultant status which saw the greatest changes.

MMC decreed that having gained their medical degree, doctors were to work in jobs gaining general medical experience (foundation programme) for two years designated as FY1 and FY2, during which time they would be granted full registration. So the old pre-registration house officer post had effectively been extended from one year to two years. During this initial two-year period doctors had to make their choice as to which career they wished to pursue and make the appropriate application.

If their choice was general practice, they would apply for a three year-training scheme and – on successful completion – they would receive a CCT which permitted them to practise as a GP.

Likewise, if the doctor chose to train in a hospital specialty such as surgery or paediatrics, they would apply for an appropriate training scheme as a specialist registrar (StR) following foundation training. Taking surgery as an example, the period required in training as an StR is six years. (The time in StR training varies from specialty to specialty between five to eight years.) On completion, the CCT is granted and the doctor is eligible to apply for a post as a consultant. The StR training is more strictly orchestrated and inflexible than in the old system. The curriculum and assessment is standardised throughout the country by means of the Postgraduate Medical Education and Training Board. I repeat that I am puzzled at the notion that reduced time and experience in training of consultants benefits patients or the health service. Or indeed the consultant. As for the standardisation of training experience throughout the country, I suppose there are arguments either way. It is salutary to note that according to the Tooke Report (2008) only 1% of doctors surveyed believed that the MMC changes would benefit clinical care given to patients, while 58% believed patients would receive no benefit.

The training aspect of the MMC changes apart, the scheme required a wholesale reorganisation of all the junior hospital jobs in the health service and arrangements for the appointments to these posts. In time gone by, a doctor would look through the advertisements and choose to apply for a job which suited his or her career aspirations and was located in a part of the country they wished to live. To complement the new MMC training system, the Medical Training Application Service (MTAS) was set up to coordinate applications for training posts nationally and allocate doctors to these posts. The system proved a shambles, not least because only 18,500 training posts were made available for the 32,000 doctors who were applying for them, leaving 13,500 doctors without a job. Unsurprisingly, there was much voluble disquiet amongst junior doctors and resignations from senior doctors who felt that their advice and warnings had been ignored. MTAS threw in the towel and handed over the application process to the medical royal colleges and local medical school deaneries.

The effect on the morale of young doctors was catastrophic. Rather than making the career pathway simpler and more efficient, MMC achieved the precise opposite. The chaotic introduction of the new scheme left thousands of doctors with no job or training post and the stress and anguish heaped upon many of them was enormous. Again, it is difficult to see how this state of affairs could have assisted in achieving the stated aim of improving the delivery of clinical care to patients.

So, what were the reasons for the changes? My honest opinion is that part of the reason was – as happens more often in government than is generally realised –

the government decided to make the changes... because it could. Another important consideration was that the changes were consistent with a philosophy that was being pursued concurrently by government through the GMC. To reinforce the notion that doctors were no longer an independent profession, largely able to govern themselves and decide their own futures, the jobs in which they were employed and the hospitals in which they worked but were now under the control of the government and its agents. MMC was essentially the final revocation of the deal that Bevan had made with the doctors at the outset of the NHS, that he was not going to turn doctors into government employees. The final nail in the coffin. From now on doctors were to be directed and cajoled at every turn by the government. The notion of an independent medical profession was well and truly dead.

CHAPTER 7

The Physician Associate

"The whole point of this system is to allow non-medically qualified people to do the job of a doctor, but claim they are not" ***@Burnt2020 on Twitter***

In Chapter 4 I described how the fundamental purpose of the 1858 Medical Act was to produce a register of properly trained medical professionals who were legally allowed to practise as doctors. Thus, the population could be sure they were being treated by someone who had been trained to do the job and had passed the requisite exams at medical school – and certainly not being treated by a quack. The GMC retained this admirable doctrine for 166 years. Until 2024 in fact, when, to fall in line with government policy, almost certainly against the better judgement of the medical profession as a whole, and with the man and woman in the street largely oblivious to what was happening, the GMC chose to register people who had not studied for five years at Medical School, and had not passed the rigorous qualifying exam at the end of it to be awarded a degree in medicine. I refer to the so-called Physician Associate.

So what exactly is a Physician Associate (PA)? The concept grew up in the US military in WW2. A cut down medical course was introduced to produce medics rapidly as they were needed in the war effort. The term in those days was actually Physician Assistant. After the war the grade evolved and became part of civilian practice. Other countries introduced a similar grade of PA though their training and scope of practice varied significantly from country to country. The first PAs were introduced into the NHS in England in 2005. Ostensibly the role of the PA, at that stage, was by no means as controversial as it was later to become. Their role was intended to relieve doctors of routine procedures and administration thereby increasing efficiency by letting doctors get on with doctoring proper. PAs were allowed to examine and suggest treatment plans for patients, supposedly along strictly defined protocols, and only under the constant supervision of a qualified doctor. They were not allowed to prescribe drugs or order tests involving ionising radiation (X-rays in other words). The concept was very much that of a doctor's assistant – hence the name physician assistant.

The problem which developed was that the NHS authorities soon – cynically – saw an opportunity with the PA grade to obtain doctor substitutes on the cheap. The practice guidelines for PAs became honoured as much in the breach as in the observance. This was to reach the stage whereby – in general practice – patients were being seen, examined, diagnosed and treated by PAs without ever seeing a qualified doctor. The most shocking thing about this was that patients being seen by a PA in general practice almost invariably believe they are being seen by a qualified doctor when they are not. In some cases, patients have been wilfully misled as to what grade of practitioner they have consulted. When a patient goes to their GP surgery and is ushered into a consulting room and sees before them someone sitting at a desk with a stethoscope draped over their shoulders – the natural assumption is that this is a qualified doctor and the patient never dreams of checking what sort of person they are seeing. At the time of writing there are approximately 3,500 PAs employed by the NHS, and the government plans to increase the numbers to 10,000 over the next ten years. The majority of PAs are employed in general practice.

It might be helpful to outline the training of a PA and compare it with that of a doctor. To become a PA, candidates need to complete a two-year MSc in Physician Associate Studies. There are at present 40 universities in the UK offering these courses. Entry requirement on to the course is normally via a degree in a life science. There is flexibility, however (and one entrant at least was accepted on to the PA course through a degree in English literature). Course entry can also be obtained through other qualifications such as in nursing or midwifery. Incidentally, the one group specifically banned from training as a PA are – wait for it – qualified doctors! Over the two-year course 1600 hours of clinical training are given, which approximates to 16 hours per week, on average, over the duration of the course. This includes general medicine, mental health, surgery and paediatrics. Much training is on a remote or virtual basis. One criticism is that so little time is spent in clinical training spread over several specialties that it is very difficult to obtain much practical experience in any of them. At the end of the course there is a qualifying exam. Pass rates are high – the University of Brighton quotes 100% on its website – which suggests, to me at least, that the exam cannot be very searching if nobody fails it. After their two-year training course the PA is able to apply for a job in the NHS, in hospital or general practice.

So, how does the training of a PA compare with medical training proper? There are 46 medical schools in the UK where students can study for a medical degree. The academic requirements are high and – to gain entry to Medical School – entrants typically have to score AAA at A level. Training is over five years. On graduating, the doctor is awarded the combined degrees of Bachelor of Medicine, Bachelor of Surgery (usually written as MB ChB or MB BS or a variant thereof) together with a provisional licence to practise. She (female doctors are now the majority) or he next has to complete two years of supervised work in medicine and surgery (Foundation Training) during which time the doctor will have gained full registration with the GMC provided their performance is signed off as adequate. So, seven years down the line from entering medical school our tyro is now qualified to... undertake further training!

On completing the foundation course, the doctor has to decide if they want to become a GP or follow a career in hospital medicine in the hope of eventually becoming a consultant. The former requires a further three years' work/training in hospital and general practice which, if successful, leads to the issuing of a CCT (Certificate of Completion of Training) allowing the doctor to practise independently as a GP. So, after 10 years we have our GP. In fact, many GPs go on to do extra training to allow them to do a limited amount of specialist work such as obstetrics.

If the doctor, on completing foundation training, wants to become a hospital consultant, the training is even longer. The exact time depends on the specialty. For example, to become a general surgeon requires another six years' training in hospitals, and exams, before a CCT can be issued. So, that's a minimum of 13 years since starting medical school. In reality it may take rather longer because to achieve one of the sought after posts in a major university hospital will require additional qualifications such as completing a doctoral thesis based on a period of scientific research. So:

- Ten years to become a qualified GP.
- 13 years to become a qualified surgeon.
- Two years to become a Physician Associate.

I believe these figures speak for themselves. Does it matter? I believe it does because PAs are routinely being used as substitutes for doctors. NHS grandees will deny this but the facts are self-evident.

In the hospital setting PAs have been used to cover registrar on-call rotas. The patient usually does not know they are not being seen by a qualified doctor. In some instances even the nurses on the ward are not aware that the individual on the registrar on-call rota is not a qualified doctor. There are even documented instances of PAs carrying out surgery including neurosurgical procedures on the brain.

But the most extensive use of PAs is in general practice. There is ample evidence that PAs are not being used here in their intended role but as doctor substitutes unbeknown to the patients. Emily Chesterton was a 30-year-old actress who attended her GP surgery in London to see – as she believed – the doctor. In fact, she saw a PA. Emily complained of a painful calf. A sprain was diagnosed and she was recommended to take paracetamol. Shortly afterwards Emily returned to the surgery with worsening symptoms. Her leg was swollen and hot and she had become breathless. Again (and again unknowingly to her) she saw the PA. This time anxiety was diagnosed and she was prescribed a tranquilliser. Three weeks after the initial consultation Emily died of pulmonary embolus. In fact the pain in her leg was due to a blood clot or thrombosis. Untreated, the blood clot broke away and travelled up the blood vessels to her heart and lungs, causing death. It was only after this tragedy that Emily's family realised she had never been seen by a doctor. But by a PA. The coroner was highly critical of the case. Emily's mother said she was "100%" sure that if Emily had been seen by a qualified doctor she would have survived. I can fully understand why Emily's mother believes this. To any qualified doctor, the presentation of a young woman of childbearing age, likely on the pill, with a painful, swollen calf and breathlessness would set a huge red flag waving right in front of your eyes. Absolutely classic case of deep vein thrombosis and pulmonary embolism – a very well recognised condition which every qualified doctor has seen. Without urgent treatment, potentially fatal. What happened in this tragic case is exactly what was supposed not to happen with PAs. Because PAs were never meant to see, diagnose and treat undifferentiated patients which is precisely what happened here. Sadly, this is how PAs are being used in many GP surgeries around the country. As non-medically qualified substitutes for trained doctors.

Shortly before going to press (April 2025) the British Medical Association published a report containing more than 600 examples of PAs putting patients at risk. A litany of impersonating doctors, illegally prescribing medications, ordering scans and misdiagnosing cancer.

A junior doctor reported:

> *"A PA in a GP surgery saw a woman with post-menopausal bleeding and documented a normal cervical examination. She came to the clinic and had a 6cm cervical cancer".*

A consultant reported:

> *"PA is conducting ward rounds unsupervised, signing [do not attempt resuscitation orders], and covering doctors' rotas, diagnosing undifferentiated patients, prescribing medication".*

Another consultant reported:

> *"I asked for a specific patient investigation to be done immediately. I later learned my decision had been overruled by a PA, which caused a delayed diagnosis and patient harm".*

The website of a large GP medical centre in north London (not the surgery which Emily Chesterton attended) lists on its website four qualified GPs and no fewer than nine Physician Associates as working at the surgery. Various other attached staff are mentioned including nurses, healthcare assistants and pharmacists. The website lists more than 100 conditions and indicates which staff member it would be most appropriate for the patient to see for each condition. For some the GP is recommended, for others the nurse, for some the recommendation is to go urgently to A&E and so on. Not once is the recommendation that the appropriate individual the patient should see is a PA, even though PAs outnumber every other type of staff member at the surgery. Perhaps I am missing something, but which patients are the PAs seeing, therefore? As I read the website, the PA is not the recommended point of contact for any of the multiplicity of conditions listed. So why are nine PAs listed on the website? What are they doing? Though the names of the nine PAs at the surgery are listed directly beneath those of the GPs, there is no indication as to what service they actually provide at the surgery. Why is the website not more informative on this point?

Professor Andrew Elder, the president of the Royal College of Physicians of Edinburgh, penned a poignant paper in the British Medical Journal entitled "*Medicine is difficult – there are no shortcuts*". This short piece refers no fewer than 12 times to the difficulty of the discipline, with Elder writing: "*Medicine is difficult, has become more difficult over my 40-year career, and will continue to become more difficult... The visions of future healthcare that have produced this mission to generate more doctors or more 'associate professionals' in shorter and shorter timeframes [are] based on a political concept of 'productivity' that is alien to those who walk the wards, talk to patients, and see the quality of care, rather than its quantity, as paramount*".

There are financial incentives for practices to employ PAs rather than qualified GPs. It has to be emphasised that PAs are not being employed to fill posts because of a shortage of GP applicants because, at the time of writing, there are several thousand (exact estimates vary) fully trained GPs who have their CCT but cannot find a job. It is simply that it is cheaper – and made deliberately so by government incentives – for the practice to employ a PA rather than a qualified GP.

How are PAs cheaper? In simple terms there are financial incentives as to why a hospital or GP practice might prefer to employ a PA as opposed to a qualified doctor. Though, as already stated, a PA is supposed to work under the supervision of a qualified doctor and is restricted from prescribing and ordering tests exposing the patient to ionising radiation, there is abundant evidence that this restriction is flouted. Few patients being treated by – or even in some cases operated on – have the faintest idea they are not being seen by a qualified doctor. So PAs are, in practice, being used as substitutes for qualified doctors and there has been a quite remarkable attempt to construct a form of words which claims that this is not the case when it is self-evident that it is. In their recent literature even the GMC has started referring not so much to "doctors" but "medical professionals". For my own part I can only see this as a desire to obfuscate and blur the distinction between PAs and qualified doctors.

Let's look at some actual costs (2024/25 figures):

Comparing the basic salaries paid to doctors and PAs on qualification. The figure (at the time of writing in 2025) is £36,616 pa for the doctor and £37,339 for the PA. I am puzzled as to why it is that the PA is paid more after two years' training than is the doctor after five years' training.

Next, let's look at the situation of a PA with two or three years' experience since qualification compared to a doctor of the same experience since obtaining their medical degree working on a hospital surgical unit registrar on-call rota. The PA's salary is £50,224 while that of the registrar is £49,909. Again, the PA is paid more than the qualified doctor.

Looking at these salaries you might well ask the question – if PAs are being paid the same or even more than doctors – how can there be a cost saving to the NHS in employing them rather than doctors? While the salary figures quoted earlier are correct, in context, they do not take account of the training costs and the long-term career costs.

It should be self-evident that a two-year course to train a PA costs considerably less than a five-year course to train a doctor. But the real cost savings are long term. The recommended salary for an NHS GP ranges from £73,114 to £110,330 pa. So, in a 30-year career as a GP (ignoring inflation and on costs such as national insurance and pension contributions) the cost to the NHS is going to be in the order of £3 million. The maximum salary paid to a PA is currently NHS Band 7 or £52,809. So, again ignoring on-costs and inflation, the cost over a 30-year career as a PA to the NHS will be in the order of £1.5 million. Or half the cost of a GP. It is difficult to find out exactly how many of the approximately 3,500 PAs currently employed in the NHS are in general practice. But the figure is probably in excess of 2,000. The NHS plans to expand PA numbers to 10,000 over the next decade. Based on the same proportion, therefore, the saving to the NHS over a 30-year career with this expansion of the grade – by employing PAs in general practice rather than qualified doctors – would be £8.5 billion.

The growing disquiet about the role of PAs led to the new Labour government in 2024 appointing Prof Gillian Leng, a public health doctor, to collect information and lead a review into the physician associate grade. It is not clear when her report is likely to be completed and published.

CHAPTER 8

Where has this wind blown us?

The medical profession in 2025

Where we are today with the medical profession is an easy question to answer. The profession, as an independent profession, is dead. For the most part we are highly skilled technicians employed and directed by government. A strange death in that few saw it coming until it was too late, certainly not the erstwhile profession itself. When the NHS was formed in 1948, the doctors could have chosen to play a major part in making the new health service a great success. Or they could have chosen to break it to pieces before it had even got off the ground. Wisely, they chose the former. Put simply, at its commencement the NHS needed the doctors more than the doctors needed the NHS. Today, the doctors need the NHS more than the NHS needs the doctors. A complete reversal in the balance of power.

Despite their initial scepticism the doctors had soon become amongst the staunchest defenders of the nascent

NHS. They did not realise that they were opening the door to their own profession's demise should an ideologically-driven government come to power which despised the post-war consensus. In time, when a government came along which had an entirely different view about the provision of public services and an aversion to just about anything run by the state, the doctors had become so subsumed in the NHS that they were no longer able to defend themselves. No longer able to defend the best interests of their patients. The doctors had fallen into the trap of thinking that the consensus approach to the NHS by the three Labour and two Conservative governments in the post-war period would continue indefinitely. When after 30 years a government with a different philosophy came along, the doctors were ill-prepared to resist and, indeed, for a long time did not fully appreciate what was happening. Within the newly formed NHS, the doctors had, for a long time, been able to get on with their job of treating patients and not worry too much about the politics. But then the politics crept up on them and pounced when they were least expecting it.

At its inception the NHS facilitated the traditional doctor/patient relationship which had persisted for centuries. Doctors had the clinical freedom to treat their patients as they believed best. Today, the doctor works for the government and can do for his or her patients and for himself/herself only what the government permits, sanctions and directs. Bevan's promise that he was not going to turn doctors into civil servants was kept for a generation, but is now long forgotten, long scorned.

At the commencement of the NHS the medical profession maintained its own standards and career structure, was responsible for its own training, young doctors were free to choose to apply for the jobs they wanted at the hospitals of their choice. No longer. The medical profession in England today is the most heavily regulated in the world. The regulation is controlled by the government or its agents, and the concept of an independent medical profession has been all but lost.

Talking with senior medical colleagues, most accept, more or less, the thesis put forward in these pages concerning the demise of the medical profession. Younger colleagues take the view that the tipping point, when the medical profession died as an independent profession, was in 2016 when the ex-government civil servant Charlie Massey took over the GMC. What I have tried to explain in this book – as someone considerably longer in the tooth – is that the key change began much earlier, carefully planned, in the 1980s with the introduction of the Griffiths changes. Warnings were clearly given in the Weekend World programme alluded to in Chapter 1 of what was to turn out to be a stealthy, long-term plan. But, for some reason, this was not picked up on by the profession at the time. Probably explained by hubris, the doctors seemed to think their position was unassailable. After all, it had been for centuries. It was not the only mistake the profession was to make.

The journey which began in the 1980s marked by Griffiths was not primarily an anti-doctor agenda as such. The doctors were simply seen as one obstacle in one area which needed to be overcome to allow the introduction of a new all-encompassing political philosophy which was to extend over all aspects of national life and ultimately become the driving force behind both of our major political parties. Neoliberalism. It wasn't just doctors. In other areas miners, steelworkers, teachers, local councils and many other groups were similarly seen as political obstacles to be crushed by the juggernaut.

One of the reasons the doctors were caught napping in the 1980s was the wrong assumption that the post-war consensus about the nature of the NHS between alternating Labour and Conservative governments was sacrosanct. The health service had been brought about in order to improve healthcare. That was its primary purpose, and governments had knuckled down to fund it appropriately. In the first 30 years and more of its existence, the NHS had largely fulfilled that role. It wasn't perfect. Nothing is. But in these terms it was doing what it was supposed to do. Therefore there was no great clamour for fundamental change. The NHS was not seen to be failing in its stated primary purpose of improving the health of the nation. What became different under Thatcher was that the NHS's success in providing clinical care for patients no longer became the primary concern for government. The primary issue was to make everything fit into a new political philosophy, one which was actually at complete odds with the philosophy under which the NHS had been originally set up, and under which it had operated more or less successfully for a generation. Prof Elder's remark quoted in the previous chapter that it was now the quantity of healthcare, rather than its quality, which had become the important thing for government, rings so very true.

It may be helpful to compare the lot of a young doctor obtaining his or her medical degree from an English university today compared to what it was like for me when I graduated in the 1970s. The first thing to say is that it is unlikely that I would have been in a position to go to medical school in the first place had I been born 50 years later in the post-Thatcher, post-Blair world. Coming from a working-class family living on a northern council estate there is no way I or my family could have afforded the tuition fees or paid for my accommodation and maintenance. Yet, with the grant system as it was then, I was able to receive an education, paid for by the state, allowing me to become, in time, a London teaching hospital consultant and my brother to become a medical school professor. In my anatomy dissection group of four students during my first term at medical school, three of us came from working class backgrounds. There was no question of loans or interest payments or taking jobs during term time. (There was in fact only one student in my year who did have a part-time job which she was able to fit in with her studies. The young lady in question had exceptionally long, elegant legs and she worked as a model, modelling tights and stockings.)

If someone wanting to become a doctor today were fortunate enough to obtain the requisite high academic grades to win a place at medical school, and to successfully navigate the various interviews and aptitude tests (which for good or ill didn't exist in my day) they would be faced with tuition fees and maintenance grants which were unknown when I was a student. The thought of ending up with a debt of up to £100,000 on graduation, to be paid off, with interest, is a game changer when deciding on a career. Undoubtably this puts off young people, who might well make excellent doctors, but who come from less privileged backgrounds, from applying to medical school. In other words, the present system militates against those from working class backgrounds to a much greater extent than in my day. Many students now take on jobs during term time to boost their income, in many instances just to survive. Typically these jobs are in the hospitality industry, working in the evenings in pubs and restaurants. I knew two medical students personally in London who worked as strippers in (so-called) gentleman's clubs. It seems to me that working in the evenings like this cannot be helpful to one's studies, at least not in a vocational degree like medicine. During my clinical years I really was on the wards, in the operating theatre, Casualty department (as A&E was called then), post-mortem room, lecture theatre or wherever gaining experience throughout the day and often at weekends. Having to work every evening in a pub or restaurant would have been an unwelcome distraction at best and potentially exhausting at worst. Of course, there are those who are simply not in a position to take on a job while studying at university, for example, those with family responsibilities. My brother describes the case of a young single mother he tried to help as her tutor. She was a very good student, who would have made an excellent doctor, but because of her childcare responsibilities as a single mother simply could not take on an evening job so could not afford to continue with the course. So the funding system which, ironically was accelerated under a Labour government led by Blair, has served to make it more difficult for people such as those from a working-class background and with family responsibilities to go to medical school. Is this really what we want?

As already described in Chapter 6, when I graduated in the 1970s you could simply apply for any house job anywhere you liked and the chances are you would get it. If you didn't get your first choice, you would very likely get your second. I don't know anyone in my circle of friends at medical school who didn't get the pre reg house job they wanted. There were enough jobs for everyone. Today, the young doctor has to go through a lengthy application process where allocations are made on what appears to be an unfathomable basis. Although doctors are allowed five choices of the jobs they would like, many end up being allocated to none of them. All entirely unsatisfactory. Young doctors may end up being posted to jobs at short notice as to where in the country they are being sent. Sudden house or flat moves may be required, uprooting of family, all very inconvenient – and very stressful.

Regarding speciality training, in my day I simply applied for the jobs I wanted at the hospitals I wanted, working for the consultants I preferred. Most of the time I got the job I wanted. If not, I certainly got a perfectly acceptable second choice. The system worked well. For the most part the system suited the junior doctors and the senior doctors for whom they worked and who trained the juniors. You chose the jobs which you felt would give you the broadest training and experience in your chosen specialty.

Specialist training for the young doctor today is so much more prescriptive, inflexible and standardised throughout the country. Applications are through an NHS software system called Oriel. Put simply, there are fewer training posts available than doctors applying for them so that there is uncertainty for many homegrown doctors that there is a future for them at all in the NHS. To further add insult to injury, young doctors today have to pay the exam fee for the examinations essential to progress in training and the associated expenses. In my day the exam fee, associated travel and subsistence expenses were reimbursed by the health authority. It is not surprising that there is a growing exodus of UK doctors abroad, despairing of the situation at home, especially to Australia and New Zealand.

Another issue with current training of hospital specialists is, as mentioned several times already, despite all the regimentation and sophisticated digitalisation, that doctors acquire significantly less practical experience on completing specialist training than in my day. As stated in Chapter 6, whereas an average of 21,000 hours' training was required to produce a consultant in the old system the new system means consultant status can be achieved with as little as 6,000 hours' training. Hence allegations that more consultants are being produced by "dumbing down". Something else which has served to restrict experience gained in training was the implementation in the UK of the European Working Time Regulation which restricted doctors' on-call hours. A report from the Association of Surgeons in Training stated that 65 hours of work per week, to include on-call and emergency cover was necessary for adequate specialist training. But the European directive did not allow such out of hours experience to be gained.

CHAPTER 9

The failure of the medical profession

In order to get to grips with the changes in the NHS and regulation and training of the medical profession over the past 40 years it is necessary to consider the record of the medical profession itself. This is an aspect which tends to be underplayed by doctors. The notion that doctors themselves have been complicit in the decline of their own profession – or, at best, failed to resist the encroachment – is something little discussed within the profession. None of this is meant to excuse the behaviour of the politicians, or to blame the state we are in today exclusively on the doctors, but it is meant to highlight a failure of senior doctors – doctors' leaders if you will – to resist harmful changes to the NHS and medical training in the way they could have done – and in my view should have done. I don't believe the doctors could have – or should have – resisted every change just for the sake of it. But they could have played a rather less passive and rather more proactive and constructive role in developments than they actually have.

There is a paradox in medicine which, I suspect, is mirrored in other professions and walks of life. There is the doctor who gets on with their job, may be totally absorbed in it and does not bother themselves with the surrounding politics. At the other extreme there is what used to be described by colleagues as "a good committee man" that is a doctor who deliberately seeks out administrative and advisory appointments (known somewhat cynically by colleagues as "gong hunters"). I can remember several examples of senior consultants who spent the majority of their time away at the royal colleges and a host of other committees of various sorts so that you hardly ever saw them in their hospital. The paradox is that the doctors who spend most time involved with their patients – whom you would acknowledge are better placed to know how the system is functioning – are not always the ones who give advice to government about the needs of the service.

The experience I had in my early years as a consultant in London sticks in my mind. It was at the time the Griffiths changes were being introduced. The health authority in which I worked contained two general hospitals, a children's hospital, a maternity hospital, a hospital which served as a long stay unit for care of the elderly and mental health services, and a handful of smaller specialist community clinics. The health authority proposed to close all five hospitals and replace them with one hospital encompassing all the general and specialist services. The upshot was that 1,100 in-patient beds in the part of inner London covered by the health authority would be lost to gain 600 beds in the new hospital. In other words, almost half their patient beds would be lost at a stroke inevitably impacting adversely on the provision of hospital care in the locality. The plan did go ahead and was completed surprisingly quickly. At the time I happened to have good contacts both with the Regional Health Authority and Westminster. The driving force behind this particular plan was twofold. First, the closed hospitals were to be sold off to the private sector for residential development (land values in this part of London being astronomical) which they were. The idea was that the money from the sale was returned to the NHS. Whether it ever was, or not, I have no idea. What is clear is that private developers made a killing. The second part of the plan was that the closures would require fewer doctors (and other staff), thus saving money on salaries. It was predicted that older consultants reluctant to be involved in the upheaval would elect for early retirement. The younger consultants would remain, enthused to work at a brand new university teaching hospital. Two birds with one stone. The older consultants, traditionally more politically powerful, organised, and obstructive to change, would be gone. It would be much easier for management to deal with the new, young consultants, somewhat inexperienced in the ways of the world and naive.

Although the first part of the plan – the land sales – seemed to go as planned, the second part did not. The reduced NHS facilities and workload meant that the senior consultants had an easier life with less work to do in the NHS and thus more time to spend at their lucrative private practices, which they did. There was no incentive for them to retire, quite the opposite. They were being paid a protected salary and protected pension contributions for doing less work. Hardly surprising that all chose to stay on and none retired even a year or two early. The younger consultants, with the drive and enthusiasm of youth, were in a position to move on to pastures new, not tied down by an established private practice, and many did so, mistrustful of the Health Authority's ruthless disregard for the provision of services. I was one of them.

The shenanigans surrounding this health authority development plan will live with me forever. Despite much vocal disquiet about the plan in the local community – concerns about the loss of local hospitals and massive reduction in bed numbers – there was very little resistance from the consultants. I do not know the exact figure but there must have been in excess of a hundred consultants from all the specialties working in the group. Of these, only six (of which I was one), spoke out against the changes and joined in action which the local community attempted to mobilise to resist the closures. There is no doubt that some colleagues were offered inducements to come on board with the plan. One close colleague told me he was "promised" he would succeed to a prestigious university professorial chair if he co-operated. (He did co-operate. The hospital closures went ahead. He was not, however, subsequently appointed to the chair.) I know what I was offered: to take a two-year sabbatical working anywhere in the world I wanted on full pay with expenses. Then come back when all the changes had gone through. A good way of getting me off the scene for a while after which time, when I returned, everyone would have forgotten who I was. I declined the offer. All the same, the Health Authority was successful in getting rid of me anyway because, when it became clear that the development was unstoppable, I resigned and moved on elsewhere. Having opposed the project in the way I had, I could not see how I could become part of it.

As already remarked, very few of my consultant colleagues stood with me in opposing the hospital closures. Of the older consultants the view seemed to be – does it really matter? It's going to happen anyway no matter what we do. It will mean less work for me and greater opportunities for private practice. Fine. Let it roll. A number of newly appointed consultants, while concerned about the likely adverse impact of the changes, were simply too frightened to rock the boat in case doing so impacted adversely on their careers in the future.

This episode brought home to me for the first time that the senior medical profession, once the scourge of governments, had become supine. I remember pointing out at the time that if the profession did not stand up against the government which was clearly hell bent on undermining the NHS, we would reach the stage where it was too late and the government would realise it could do with the medical profession pretty much as it wished. This is, in my view, exactly what was to happen. My colleagues let it happen.

There were – and are – a number of doctors' organisations purporting to represent the views of their members. Typically, each specialty or sub speciality has its own professional club. There are many dozens of them. But there are two organisations of particular note: the BMA (British Medical Association) and the Royal Colleges. Regarding the latter, there are 14 Royal Colleges based in the United Kingdom. The oldest of these – the Royal College of Surgeons of Edinburgh and the Royal College of Physicians of London – were founded in the 16th century. Some colleges – like the Royal College of General Practitioners and the Royal College of Ophthalmologists – are much more recent. Traditionally the royal colleges maintained standards and oversaw training in their respective disciplines. Admission to the membership or fellowship of a royal college signified that a high level of professional competence had been achieved. For a senior doctor to be elected on to the governing council of a royal college by his peers was seen within the profession as achieving great status. Becoming president of a royal college even more so, often leading to the award of a knighthood or DBE.

With the formation of the NHS the royal colleges did not become the arm of the medical profession responsible for negotiating with the government. Unsurprising, as none of them represented the profession as a whole or claimed to. Nevertheless, if they wished to put forward a point of view to the government on behalf of their fellows' and members' specialist interests, they would certainly do so. The government would be unlikely to ignore them, in the early years of the NHS at least.

The role of representing the profession as a whole to the government fell to the BMA. The BMA long predated the NHS, having been founded in 1836. By the time of the NHS not all doctors were members of the BMA, but most were, whether GP, surgeon, pathologist, radiologist or whatever. There was even a section for medical students. The BMA was effectively the doctor's trade union and was formally registered as such in 1971. The BMA was an important and influential organisation and publishes one of the most prestigious medical journals in the world – the British Medical Journal. In the early years of the NHS, the general secretary of the BMA was a figure of national importance. I well remember that when I was a sixth former and medical student the general secretary was Dr Derek Stevenson. He was always popping up on the TV news. It says something about the fall from prominence of the BMA that I myself did not know the name of the present head of the BMA until I looked it up.

A unique function of the BMA at the introduction of the NHS was to conduct pay and contract negotiations with the government on behalf of doctors. It was through the BMA's prolonged negotiations with Bevan at the inception of the NHS that doctors achieved payment by capitation fee for GPs and pay beds in NHS hospitals for consultants. In the 1960s pressure from the BMA led to the setting up of an independent review body to decide doctors' pay. The biggest dispute between the BMA and government up to that time was the junior doctors' strike in 1975/76. This was a bad tempered, drawn out affair which eventually resulted in what was at least a partial victory for the doctors. The next major confrontation with the government over pay and contracts was another junior doctors' dispute which began in 2015. This was even more bad tempered and drawn out than the one 40 years earlier. The basis of the dispute was the desire of the Health Secretary Jeremy Hunt to impose a new contract on junior doctors after negotiations had got nowhere. As a consequence, a ballot organised by the BMA amongst junior doctors produced a remarkable 98% vote in favour of strike action. The strikes did go ahead. The doctors had significant support amongst the population at large. It should also be noted that the junior doctors had the support of most of their senior colleagues in 2015, something which was not always evident in 1975. There were unprecedented marches and demonstrations with celebrity endorsements. There is little doubt that, in an earlier age, given the backing the juniors had, they would have been successful in the dispute. But things had changed. The government held firm. Hunt was not going to be intimidated or browbeaten by the doctors. This was the clearest indication to date that – when it came to the balance of power between the government and the medical profession – the boot was well and truly on the other foot. In 2016 the doctors took the government to court, arguing that it was unlawful for Hunt to impose the new contract unilaterally. The court ruled that Hunt did have the power to do so. The doctors called off their industrial action though the dispute itself remained unsettled and dragged on until the election of a Labour government in 2024 when a new contract was finally agreed.

Nothing in the history of the NHS exacerbated the bad feeling on the part of the doctors towards the government as much as the 2015 dispute. It wasn't solely the pay and contract issue. The ongoing changes to training and career structure were causing much stress and unhappiness. There was a breakdown in trust with the government. There was a realisation that the medical profession was now largely powerless in a confrontation with the government, whether backed by the BMA or not. To put it bluntly, the government had demonstrated it could do pretty much as it liked with doctors and there was nothing the doctors could do about it.

While the BMA served to negotiate contract terms, conditions of service and pay with the government on behalf of the profession as a whole, the royal colleges' interest was in maintaining standards of competence and training within their specialties. Any concerns or recommendations pertaining to these matters could be conveyed to government. For many years – and this was the case when I was a junior doctor in training in the late 1970s and early 1980s – the major role of the royal colleges was to issue, following a vigorous and testing examination, a diploma certifying the holder had reached a certain level of competence in the specialty, allowing them to proceed to the final stage of training to become a consultant. In each case this led to a postnominal much coveted by doctors in training (such as MRCP – Member of the Royal College of Physicians, or MRCOG – Member of the Royal College of Obstetricians and Gynaecologists and so on). Later in the 1980s the Colleges began to issue certificates of higher professional training – based on experience acquired rather than by examination – indicating that a doctor had reached the required level of experience and competence to become a consultant.

Unlike the BMA, the royal colleges were not traditionally in regular conflict with the government. In my view, until relatively recently their approach was to keep the government at arm's length. It would be correct to say, I believe, that when a royal college did choose to express an opinion publicly it fairly reflected the feeling of its members and fellows. Relatively recently, however, this seemed to change over one issue in particular, with one college at least – that is the introduction of PAs into the health service (see Chapter 7).

Shortly after their introduction into the NHS, the Royal College of Physicians of London agreed in 2015 to set up a Faculty within the College for Physician Associates (or Physician Assistants as they were then called) together with a voluntary register of PAs. This did not lead to much concern initially. First, because the grade of PA was no means as controversial in those days as it was to become. Second, because there were very few PAs about anyway and few college fellows had any direct experience of them. With time the numbers of PAs began to grow, and the word "assistant" was dropped from their title in favour of "associate". It also became apparent that the role which PAs were actually being used for was rather more involved than people had been led to believe at the outset. Members of the college began to express disquiet that the college had become associated with PAs in the way it had. A survey of members was held, following which there were accusations that the college council had misrepresented the view of members consulted to imply that there was more support for the college's involvement in the PA project than there actually was. An increasing number of senior members began to question whether it was prudent for the college to be involved with PAs at all given the increasing concerns surrounding the grade. There were also accusations that the prime motivation for setting up the faculty had been financial in that it would bring more money into the College through subscriptions. The arguments became so heated that, in 2024, only the third emergency meeting of fellows was called in the college's 500-year history. This led to multiple resignations of senior officers including the president. Quite where the college now stands on the PA issue is not clear. Hopefully, the college will reach its final position on the matter when the results of the study currently being carried out by Professor Gillian Leng into the role of PAs becomes available.

In passing, the Royal College of Physicians seems to have got itself into quite a mess recently, the PA ructions apart. The College announced in 2025 that 222 doctors were incorrectly told they had passed the MRCP exam taken in 2023 which they had actually failed. A further 61 were told they had failed when in actual fact they had passed. The exam is absolutely key in training, allowing the doctor to continue to the final stage of training to become a consultant. The ramifications of this error are enormous. Professor Philip Banfield of the BMA said:

"Failing an exam is devastating and has consequences for doctors as they work their way up the ladder of expertise; being told you have failed when in fact you have passed, is even worse. For those 222 doctors who have spent the past 18 months believing they had passed, but have not, they will be equally devastated and unsure what lies ahead. The moral, legal and governance aspects of this truly terrible mistake are far-reaching and must not be under-estimated by the public, Government, and the NHS."

The PA controversy has also shaken up proceedings at the Royal College of General Practitioners. A paper published in the College's journal in 2015 by Drennan et al was broadly supportive of the introduction of PAs into general practice. It should be stated that there were very few PAs actually working in general practice at that stage and experience of them was strictly limited. There was enthusiasm that the grade might well be beneficial in relieving increasingly overworked GPs with routine and administrative tasks on a supervised basis. Consequently, the College stated its position on PAs in 2017, which was broadly supportive. There was certainly no groundswell from the College membership against. As PAs were gradually introduced into general practice and doctors became more familiar with them, concerns did start to be expressed, increasingly voluble over the years. The culmination in 2024 was that the College council voted two to one against having PAs work in general practice. A stark reversal in the College's position brought about by the experience of disgruntled members. The RCGP

President Professor Kamila Hawthorne went on to state publicly that there was "*no role*" for Physician Associates in general practice. The revised position was a great embarrassment to the government.

All credit to the royal colleges for standing up for their beliefs. All credit to the college memberships for beginning to take a stand against PAs when some might argue that the college grandees had too readily accepted government policy without fully digesting the implications. The recent events described above show that when pushed by their members – the doctors actually working at the coal face rather than sitting in a boardroom in London with a brass gong round their neck scouring the Times for the publication of the latest honours list – can mobilise their royal colleges effectively. Too often, in my view, the royal colleges appear to have seen themselves as facilitators of government policy before fully considering the impact on their members and, indeed, their members' patients. It further appears to me that the colleges' response to the government takeover of the profession over the past generation has been to encourage their members to accept government proposed changes and adapt to them as best they can rather than protesting to the government when changes were unlikely to help either the doctor or the patient.

I know that many in the college hierarchy take the view that their role is not political and they should not be challenging government policy. This is fair enough, as far as it goes, but there must come a point when for the sake of the wellbeing of both doctors and their patients it is right and proper for the College to take a stand and point out, forcefully if necessary, when proposed changes to the health service, doctors' training or whatever are bound to have adverse consequences. In many ways the royal colleges are well placed to do this, rather more so than the BMA, because the latter is essentially a trade union more often than not arguing about pay, whereas the royal colleges are highly respected learned bodies concerned with maintaining proper professional standards and adequate training of doctors. In terms of speaking up for doctors, the royal colleges are really the most authoritative voices the doctors have. I believe they should have been more vocal over the years in challenging government policies which threatened to make things worse rather than better. Admittedly they may still have failed in the face of a determined government onslaught. But they could have tried.

I suppose we are all, to a large extent, the products of our environment. The environment in which the medical profession worked before the foundation of the NHS was very different from what it was to become over the first 30 years of the NHS's existence. The environment evolved further during the second half of the NHS's existence. It is this change in environment which has, I believe, impacted so much on how the medical profession sees itself today. To someone who has spent well over 40 years in the profession, it is striking how different is the mindset of the typical doctor (if we can accept such a notion) today from when I set out on my lifetime's journey. Junior doctors today see themselves as one cog in a huge machine, very reluctant – fearful almost – of being seen to have independent thought. When I started out, young doctors had a self-confidence, in a few cases bordering on arrogance, which has totally been lost today. It could be argued that it is a good thing that this is no longer the case. I don't think it is quite so straightforward. There are swings and roundabouts and I think what has been lost is the ability for junior doctors to speak up for themselves, for their careers and ultimately for their patients.

The same is true for senior doctors, the consultants and GPs. If a newly appointed consultant wants to progress their career, work with the best personnel and facilities, the best way of doing this today is by keeping your head down. The downside of this is that there may be a tendency to attempt to secure your own little kingdom in the short term and overlook more widespread issues which may impact adversely in the long term. Dismiss them as someone else's problem. I think one of the best recent examples of this relates to the thorny issue of PAs (discussed at some length in Chapter 7). Many junior doctors are genuinely puzzled at why it is their consultants are not more critical of the PA grade and in some cases positively supportive of it. The juniors do not understand why their senior colleagues are letting them lose out in terms of training and experience in favour of a non-medical grade. The reason is that the consultant may see the PA, a permanent grade who gets to know the unit well, and the consultant's foibles and preferences, as the "glue" which holds the unit together year after year. A continuing presence, consistency in a world where junior medical staff now rotate round every few months so that by the time they become familiar with the unit they're whisked away elsewhere and replaced by another junior beginning at square one. In this respect day-to-day life is easier for the consultant with the PA. As for the junior staff who are not getting the training and experience they expect and deserve... well that's their tough luck, not the consultant's. The problem here is, of course, the inadequacies of the training programme for junior doctors in its present format, discussed earlier in this book. This produces uncertainty and instability for the juniors which, as it seems to suit the government's cause very well, the government is unlikely to seek to change.

CHAPTER 10

The Future?

"It's difficult to make predictions, especially about the future".
Mark Twain

Regarding the NHS, the recent election of a new Labour government has, as was almost inevitable, led to an announcement of a further review into the workings of the health service. Quite where this will take us and precisely what changes are in store is difficult to predict but one major change has already been announced. This is the abolition of the highest tier of NHS management, NHS England.

Given that the new administration in Westminster is wedded to the same neoliberal economic agenda as governments of both colours over the past 40 years, there is likely to be more of the same. In trying to work out likely developments it is salutary to consider that if the NHS did not exist today no politician would ever dream of creating it in anything like its present format and certainly not in the format of 1948. In a recent debate in the House of Commons Labour MP Clive Lewis stated: "*My party today would not create the NHS*". Neither would any other major party. Over the past 40 years Thatcherite neoliberal economics have prevailed and become unassailable.

Before I started writing this book, beginning to research, mulling over personal experience and talking with colleagues, I had it in my mind that those who rule over us foresaw a progression over the years to what amounts to a fully privatised health service. By this I mean a service provided by a series of large private companies running hospitals and surgeries providing services through individual health insurance policies. Most likely the insurance premiums would be means tested so that high earners paid in full whereas the poorest in society would have their premiums paid as a state benefit. Employers might well see providing health insurance to their employees as an attractive benefit to improve recruitment. While I still see this as the politicians' ultimate goal, I now believe that a fully privatised health service is still a long way off. This is not because there are not neoliberal zealots who drool at the prospect, but because most senior politicians today regard the NHS as a unique oddity in the public service spectrum, one which unlike gas, electricity, water and the railways cannot easily be privatised in the same way. Not because many would not like to, allowing their business backers to secure enormous profit; not because of any moral commitment to ensuring healthcare for all on an equitable basis; not even because of the fear of enormously negative political fallout which would be inevitable. But because it is realised that the changes would most likely increase the strain on the public purse, not reduce it. For all the talk of the free market, any savvy politician is aware that the NHS is remarkably cost efficient in providing the service it does. As long as the health service remains under government control, it is easier for politicians to keep a tight control on the narrative – and the money.

I think therefore it will be more of the same, that is gradually increasing co-operation with the private sector in an increasing number of areas of healthcare and the increasing use of private finance to fund capital projects. The current health secretary Wesley Streeting has indicated that he is sympathetic to reviving PFI-like schemes to develop infrastructure projects. It's likely that demand for health services will continue to outstrip the facilities available. I doubt there will be any motivation to significantly increase government funding to the NHS, while failing to do so will have the effect of pushing more people toward the private option. Which suits the government.

Regarding the future of the medical profession, the outlook is bleak. Once again I think we are likely to see more of the same. The government has established a whip hand over the profession, something it is not going to relinquish and something the profession is now impotent to challenge. The government now largely controls every aspect of a doctor's life and work to a quite extraordinary extent. The only realistic option left to the doctors is to vote with their feet, but there is a limit to how many of them the Australian and New Zealand health services can accommodate.

Although the medical profession is, belatedly, waking up to the dangers posed by the increasing numbers of PAs planned for the health service, and while the public is now also becoming aware of the dangers, it is likely that the experiment will accelerate for as long as the government feels able to get away with it. Recent history suggests that – when it comes to the health service – the government usually gets what it wants. It's basically taking the Thatcher/Weekend World process a stage further from emasculating the traditional medical profession to replacing it with a less highly trained group of practitioners, cheaper, more malleable and potentially much less troublesome. I can foresee a situation where patients attending for primary medical care in general practice and hospital A&E departments are routinely seen by PAs and only progress to seeing a qualified doctor having been referred on. I can also foresee the restrictions on PAs' scope of practice gradually relaxed so that their role becomes for all practical purposes indistinguishable from that carried out in the past by a qualified doctor. There will still be qualified doctors, no doubt, who will uniquely be able to rise to the senior status of a principal in general practice or a consultant in hospital. These lucky few will be the ones who are encouraged to carry out private practice – for those patients who can afford it. Or those, such as employees of the GMC, whose employer provides them with the perk of health insurance. So, we have the clear beginnings of a two-tier system whereby the well-off have access to highly trained, properly qualified doctors in the recognised meaning of the word, whereas those less fortunate have to make do with a practitioner who is not a qualified doctor and who has considerably less practical and theoretical experience. Ironically, the sombre picture described above is exactly the same unsatisfactory state of affairs as pertained prior to the Medical Act of 1858, a situation which the Act was specifically meant to remedy. We have come full circle.

CHAPTER 11

Summary and Conclusions

The evolution of the medical profession in England over several centuries is described. The 1858 Medical Act was the legislation responsible for defining the medical profession as we know it today and for setting up the GMC as the profession's regulatory body. The formation of the NHS in 1948 and its multiple revisions of management structure and organisation is outlined. The NHS has had a profound effect on the further evolution of the medical profession. The greatest impact has been the changes brought about by the Thatcher and Blair governments. There has been a significant change in the function of the GMC over the past 20 years so that it is no longer a regulatory body wholly independent of government. During the same period the democratic input of the medical profession into the GMC has been abolished.

Changes to student maintenance funding and the introduction of tuition fees have placed a massive burden on undergraduate study so that students from less advantaged social and family backgrounds are effectively discouraged from attending medical school. Financial considerations mean that students often have to take jobs when they should be studying. Students who do graduate in medicine face horrendous debts which may take decades to pay off, if ever. The newly qualified doctor is no longer able to explore and work in a number of specialities after graduation, as they choose, in order to gain broader experience before deciding on a final career choice. Postgraduate training for junior doctors has become a nightmare with uncertainty as to where they are going to work and even if there is a job available to them at all. The consultants produced at the end of today's training programme are significantly less experienced than those of a generation ago. In the environment in which they find themselves, consultants are much more inclined to pursue their own narrow interests and "keep their heads down" and avoid pointing out adverse consequences of the continuing political meddling which impacts adversely on patient care and the training of their junior colleagues.

We have come full circle since the keystone 1858 Medical Act which for 166 years, in the interests of public safety, defined who was a doctor and who was not. The GMC has abrogated that responsibility and now registers non-medically qualified individuals.

The NHS, while by no means having rotated full circle since its foundation in 1948, has turned at least through a metaphorical right angle under the stewardship of successive governments. The changes, heralded by the

Griffiths report of 1983, were not primarily concerned with the quality of care the NHS was delivering. The key concern of the government was not that the NHS was failing in its primary function of providing the best healthcare available. It clearly was not failing. Rather it was that the government resented spending money on the service. The government was no longer motivated by providing the best healthcare to its citizens but in reducing the cost of the NHS to the Treasury in the pursuit of political dogma. From its origins as an organisation which promised to facilitate the professional relationship between doctor and patient, leaving the doctor in charge of the treatment offered and promising not to turn doctors into civil servants or government employees, the NHS has gone back on both counts. The Thatcher government decided that – in order to enact the market reforms to the NHS as it wished to do – it would be necessary to undermine the power and influence of the medical profession and certainly not let the profession continue to take the lead. Having almost completely immersed itself in the NHS, the medical profession proved entirely impotent to resist government changes. A total power reversal since 1948.

As for the future, the philosophy of neoliberal economics is likely to persist no matter which party is in power. So it is likely to be more of the same. While the future of the PA grade is uncertain, and the outcome of the Leng review is awaited, whatever the recommendation it seems unlikely that the government is going to backtrack on the expansion of care provided by individuals who are not medically trained. They may change the name, they may tinker with the training schemes and job descriptions, for the sake of form, but I predict the concept is here to stay. The advantages to government in terms of keeping costs down, controlling and standardising treatment protocols and further eclipsing what residual influence the medical profession might still have, are simply seen as much too tempting to the current generation of politicians. I foresee, in time, a two-tier NHS. The better off, those with health insurance, get to see a qualified doctor. Those less well off will rely on an NHS staffed, at the first ports of call at least, with individuals whom the patient assumes is a doctor, but in reality is not.

Is this what we want? The medical profession is not in a position, today, to prevent it happening. A generation ago the profession was probably still in a position to take a stand. But for various reasons it failed to do so. That generation of senior doctors – my generation – let down the health service and the country. They let down themselves. They let down their patients.

There will be those of you who read this testimony as the somewhat soured experienced doctor at the end of his career, disillusioned, resentful that the profession in which he has worked all his life is no longer held in its traditional regard, is no longer of the same importance in the overall scheme of things as it used to be. No longer listened to. It is true that I see so much in the world that leaves me disillusioned. But I believe it would be unfair to dismiss my analysis before at least giving serious consideration to the points argued.

I have one last thing to say to you. If you are as concerned as I am by the path along which the health service appears to be travelling, for the reasons I have described and other reasons, then it really is up to you – as an ordinary citizen and voter – to speak out and try to do something about it. The politicians, despite many fine words and false smiles, will not help you. The medical profession cannot.

It really is now up to you.

EPILOGUE

"One notable academic observed that to study welfare was to highlight the values of the society within which that welfare was provided. I would argue that our values determine to a large extent what we observe."
Frank Field

In closing I seek indulgence to tell a personal story which ends in a heartfelt plea. Any doctor – especially one with a career as long as mine – will have patients he will never forget. For me, there are many. Some with uplifting stories, some with heartbreakingly sad ones. But here I relate the story of just one – because she encapsulates so much that I admire both in people as individuals and in a country to organise itself into a civilised humane society. A country and society that I, as a private citizen, can be proud to be part of and hopefully contribute to.

This is the story of (let's call her) Mary. The one thing we did know about Mary was her first name. That was consistent. As for her surname, I never knew what it was till I met her brother many years after I first got to know Mary, at Mary's funeral. She gave different surnames on different occasions at the hospital where I worked and at various other hospitals in south-west London where she was a regular attender. We never knew her date of birth. The regular receptionists knew better than to ask her age when she booked in. But a new clerk, asking this routine question in all innocence, would receive a sound scolding from Mary for asking such an impertinent, irrelevant question. My guess is that Mary was in her 80s when I first met her. We never knew if Mary had ever married, or had family. As for her address on her records, we never knew what it was. She gave a variety of different addresses, all of them in affluent areas of Chelsea or Westminster. I didn't believe any of them was correct.

Mary spent most of the day, as far as we could tell, wandering the streets with a pair of large shopping bags stuffed (I think) with old clothes. She always wore a heavy coat, scarf and thick stockings even in high summer. Persuading her to undress to be examined was a non-starter. She was a tall, elegant lady whom I imagined as a young woman – which would have been in the 1920s – would have been really quite beautiful. Indeed, her manner of speech was that of a 1920s society debutante ("Huntin', shootin', fishin'... don't cha know?") – perhaps she had been – at that time I didn't know one way or the other. Over a period of six years Mary would turn up unbooked at many of my clinics with a variety of complaints and often no complaints at all, just for a chat, in the winter to get out of the cold and perhaps a buckshee cup of tea and biscuit from the WRVS canteen if she were lucky. I would estimate I must have seen her on several hundred occasions, more often than any other patient in my long career. She would talk to me about having spent the weekend away with Lady So-and-So ("Very nice people – do you know them?") when I had seen her myself that weekend asleep on a park bench on Eelbrook Common. She would tell me about the fantastic parties she had attended and confide how concerned she was about the family works of art which had passed down to her ("original Constables and Turners") which, she assured me, she was keeping in safe storage. For some reason I never quite understood she would become quite distressed talking about these paintings because "they" were trying to take them away. I eventually deduced she meant the Revenue in lieu, I think, of family death duties.

One day, after I had known her a couple of years, Mary was brought into our hospital by emergency ambulance. Someone had found her collapsed in Battersea Park and dialled 999. She was in a poor state, drifting in and out of consciousness. She was immediately admitted to hospital under my medical colleagues for a full work up. It transpired that Mary's main problem was severe heart failure, her heart was beating irregularly and she may have had a recent myocardial infarction (heart attack). She was stabilised fairly quickly (she was, as I'd long realised, as tough as they come) and soon became quite chirpy. My colleague told me Mary was in severe heart failure owing to multiple valve disease and – if she was ever going to get mobile and out of hospital – she needed heart valve replacement surgery. To my complete surprise Mary consented to surgery without hesitation. I am no heart surgeon or cardiologist, but I did wonder if Mary would survive such a major procedure. She was transferred to the Brompton Hospital for surgery and about ten days later returned to us. I remember one afternoon I visited her between clinic and theatre list. She was blooming. She told me that she had been invited by some posh-sounding family to stay with them in Sussex to convalesce (of course, she hadn't – she hadn't had a single visitor, letter or card) and of course she hadn't been at all worried at the thought of surgery because "I know all about surgery and used to work in an operating theatre". Very good, I thought, of course you have...

When it came time for Mary's discharge (by which time she looked stronger and fitter than I had ever known her – it's amazing what a properly functioning heart can do) the social worker confirmed what I'd always suspected, that Mary was homeless. The social worker reckoned she could arrange for a council flat, but this would take some time, so she was arranging for Mary to go into sheltered accommodation until her flat was ready. I kept in touch with the social worker over Mary and, indeed, Mary was given a council flat in Westminster. Not long afterwards Mary's regular visits to my clinic started again. I was glad about this because she needed regular blood tests and blood-thinning tablets after the heart surgery (not that she ever took them) and this was an opportunity to at least try to get this right. Mary apologised for not having attended for a while explaining that "I've been staying with friends out of London – they needed help with entertaining their guests", whereas of course I knew she'd been in the sheltered hostel just down the road all the time. Over the following few years it was very much back to business as usual with Mary. She would attend my clinic every week, sometimes twice a week. She didn't like her new flat. How often she stayed there, I really don't know, but probably not very often. She basically resumed her old life. In the summer months at least she preferred the comfort of a park bench to her council flat.

I found out about Mary's death by accident. One day one of the ambulance personnel mentioned to our receptionist that the previous week they had taken Mary from a park bench in Battersea Park to another local hospital and she had been certified dead on arrival. I managed to find out the funeral details and the following week attended the funeral. She is the only patient of mine whose funeral I have ever attended. I went because she had become as much a friend as a patient and I had genuinely come to like and admire her. Someone who had chosen to live her life just the way she wanted to. But the main reason was that I was fearful that she had become so isolated that there might be no one else to attend her funeral, something that struck me as unbearably sad. In fact, the vicar apart, there were just four of us. Me, two elderly ladies who must have somehow known Mary, and Mary's younger brother whom the Social Services had managed to trace. As it turned out the only family she had.

I chatted with Mary's brother, Thomas, after the service. An unassuming man, unlike Mary he was not tall and he spoke with a distinct Geordie accent. Hardly surprising as the family came from Tyneside. Thomas told me theirs was a working class family and – as an 18 year old during the Great War – Mary had travelled south to London to enter domestic service. The family she had worked for were high society and in the last year of the war Mary had gone to France with the lady of the house to work in a field hospital before returning to Wimbledon. After that Mary had become a nanny. Mary's brother told me that in the early years after leaving home she had written regularly and on several occasions travelled north to visit family. But, over time, visits and letters had become less frequent and eventually ceased altogether. Thomas had not seen Mary for more than 30 years since their mother's funeral.

In one way I wanted to find out about Mary, but in another way I didn't want to pry into her secrets. I didn't ask her age, because it was a secret she had not wanted me to know. Thomas told me he was going round to clear out her flat, which turned out to be a small council flat near Westminster Hospital which was "*in a right state*". I mentioned that Mary had confided in me that she was very concerned about what would happen to the family's heirlooms she was holding in trust – the Constables and the Turners. Thomas laughed: "There are no paintings. Mary lived in a dream world – she has done for years."

It was all fantasy. Or was it? Mary had lived in grand houses, seen high society parties. As a domestic servant. I recalled her remark to me that she had once worked in an operating theatre. No doubt when in France in the Great War she had when she had served in a field

hospital. In her later years, as a vagrant in the streets and parks of south-west London she had affected the airs and graces of her erstwhile employers. I have no doubt that, to Mary, her world was real to her. She could have lived in no other.

So why do I tell this story? Well because it makes me incredibly proud. Why? Not because of my medical skills. My interaction with Mary was primarily social. It was the medical and surgical skills of the teams of colleagues who fixed Mary's heart who restored her to health and gave her years of active life.

And here you have it. The National Health Service. Mary had no health insurance. Nobody asked if she could pay, nobody sent her a bill. When in need she was taken from her park bench into one of the great hospitals of the world for complex cardiac surgery and – when sorted out – was ultimately allowed to return to her park bench – as was her choice. If the Queen had been admitted from Buckingham Palace she would have received identical treatment from the same people. In my opinion a National Health Service which can give identical treatment to individuals so far apart in the social strata, entirely non-judgemental, is something very special indeed.

Do not let them take it away from you. They will try.

– ENDS –

www.ingramcontent.com/pod-product-compliance
Lightning Source LLC
LaVergne TN
LVHW020235210926
848481LV00016B/2213
9781917329934